THE DUKE AND DUCHESS'S KAMA SUTRA

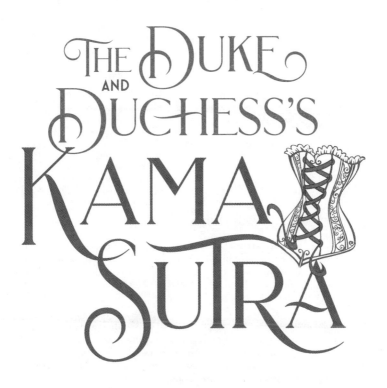

AN UNOFFICIAL BEDROOM BOOK FOR FANS OF *BRIDGERTON*

MARISA BENNETT

AUTHOR OF THE NATIONAL BESTSELLER
FIFTY SHADES OF PLEASURE

Skyhorse Publishing, Inc.

Skyhorse Publishing books may be purchased in bulk at special discounts for sales promotion, corporate gifts, fund-raising, or educational purposes. Special editions can also be created to specifications. For details, contact the Special Sales Department, Skyhorse Publishing, 307 West 36th Street, 11th Floor, New York, NY 10018 or info@skyhorsepublishing.com.

Skyhorse® and Skyhorse Publishing® are registered trademarks of Skyhorse Publishing, Inc.®, a Delaware corporation.

Visit our website at www.skyhorsepublishing.com.

10 9 8 7 6 5 4 3 2 1

Library of Congress Cataloging-in-Publication Data is available on file.

Cover design by Joanna Williams
Cover and spot illustrations courtesy of Shutterstock.com
Interior design by Joanna Williams
Illustrations by Thanos Tsilis

Print ISBN: 978-1-5107-6820-8
eBook ISBN: 978-1-5107-6974-8

Printed in the United States of America

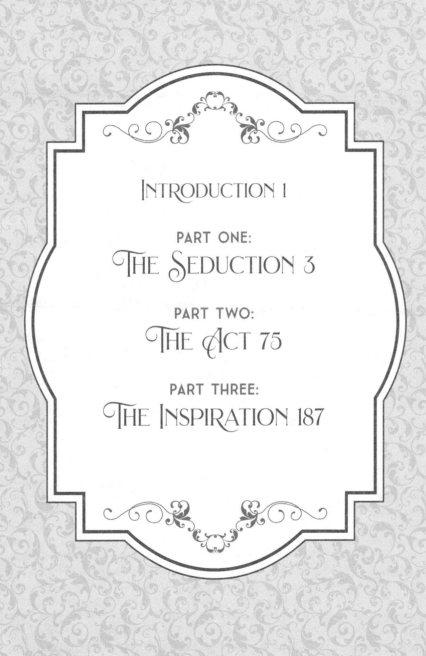

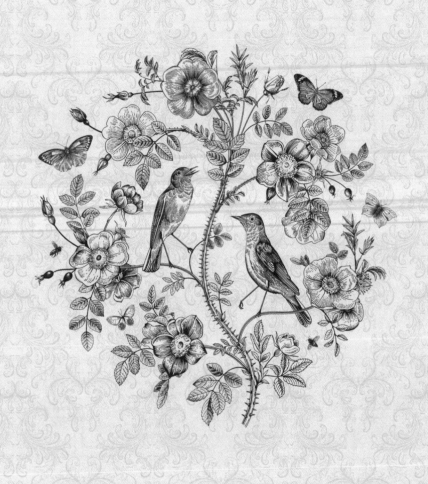

ÐEAREST READER,

SHOULD YOU HAVE FOUND your grip tightening slightly around the remote control while watching *Bridgerton*, know that you are not alone. Many a flame will be lit by the breathless glances, light caresses, and passionate embraces of Mayfair's most captivating residents. And many more roar to life with the duke's declaration of his own burning desire.

That spark has awakened in us all a longing for romance, sensual touch, uninhibited passion, and true love to rival that of the duke and duchess. With a chemistry so electric it could light all the hanging lamps at Vauxhall, the fated couple offers a great deal of inspiration, both deliciously wicked and delightfully innocent. And this author is here to reveal their steamiest secrets.

Unlike some of the more demure mamas of the *ton*, trust I shall not keep you in the dark. *The Duke and Duchess's Kama Sutra* includes intimate instructions that will make your heart race and your rouge darken. Discover tantalizing ways to tease your love, methods of self-pleasure that would make even Siena's experienced toes curl, and advice for enjoying every delectable encounter with your own rakish duke or wide-eyed duchess.

With more than fifty lusciously instructive illustrations, you will find an array of exciting ways to bring your *Bridgerton* fantasies to life. Is it the scene on the stairs that gets your blood pumping? Or perhaps the hunger in Anthony's eyes? Maybe you enjoy the innocent flirtations and solid partnerships the most. Whatever spicy scenes, dashing characters, or visual splendor set your flame alight, the ways to recreate it are at your eager fingertips!

Yours truly,

Lady Bennett

THE
SEDUCTION

GREAT EXPECTATIONS

CREATE THE COURTSHIP YOU LONG FOR in the style of Grosvenor Square's most enviable couple. Whether your own relationship is a recent betrothal, a longstanding and sturdy partnership, or a hot new flame, you can take a leaf from the duke and duchess's book—starting from the beginning. Make each encounter feel brand new by enforcing the rules of high society to build mounting desire. Subtlety and restraint are the tenets of tension for any couple of good ranking, and these courtship cues will make each stolen glance sweeter, every fleeting touch more electric, and every furtive whisper more alluring.

In the pages of this section, you will discover creative forms of flirtation to heighten anticipation, heart-racing exercises in self-discipline to make the reward worth all the wait, and tried-and-true ways to create romance and yearning that will have even the most rakish hearts melting. Open your expressive side through heartfelt love letters and enticing charcoal drawings, and learn the language of flowers to show your deepest desires through an elegant unspoken code that only you two can share. Find new ways to set a scene befitting a love like yours, relish in the small details that make your partner so enticing, and embrace self-pleasure as a form of foreplay that will make your love even more intimate.

Long for one another like never before with lessons in sensual decorum. As your romance builds and your bond deepens, you will be primed for the kind of proper romp that even the scandal sheets dare not mention. Follow along with the amorous etiquette presented ahead, and you will discover the finest ways to bring your bliss to its brim.

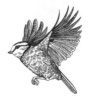

CHAPTER 1

COURTSHIP

IF THERE IS ONE THING WE SHOULD LEARN from our dear duke and duchess, it is the power of allowing your thirst for another's touch to build to thrilling heights before quenching it. In fact, that may be the sultry secret to a more fulfilling and libidinous partnership. Abiding by a few of fine society's guidelines for proper courtship can turn a natural spark into a roaring wildfire, or perhaps even fan an old flame back to life. The question is: How do you adhere to Regency rules while living in a time that considers courtship antiquated?

Truth be told, it is no one's business but your own which tools you use to stoke your own fire. If you must, imagine your tenderness and restraint as simple acts of delayed gratification, which make indulgence all the more rewarding. Read on to discover how to savor sumptuous moments, turn flirtation into art worthy of Mr. Granville's salon, cleverly tempt your partner, and test the bounds of your own propriety until your very skin is alight with yearning. When others begin to notice the fruits of your efforts, they may just follow suit!

FORGE A FRIENDSHIP

As Simon wisely states, friendship is something far greater than romance. Acting on attraction alone may be easy, but without affection, you may find yourself feeling unfulfilled. Setting aside attraction in favor of forging true friendship with your partner can lead to more explosive encounters later. To paraphrase Queen Charlotte, friendship is the best possible foundation a relationship can have. It leads to the kind of trust, adventurousness, fondness, and levity that make romantic entanglements exponentially more enjoyable.

When you are with your love, take the time to truly enjoy each other's company. Converse about your greatest desires, laugh together at the absurdity of the things (and people) around you, indulge your sweet tooth together over colorful biscuits and creamy desserts. It may be a bit simpler for our *Bridgerton* friends, with little but their embroidery to divert them, but do attempt to be present with your partner. Doing so may help you take special note of your love's more alluring qualities, like the seductive way they lick a spoon. You never know when that knowledge may prove useful!

ENTIRELY ENAMORED

The nerves of new love are certainly not to be discounted in their aphrodisiac-like effects. Simply hearing your lover's name said aloud is enough to thrill you. Their smile seems catching, and you find yourself feeling passionate about even their most irritating attributes. If you are a newly attached couple, take the time to savor the dopamine flooding your system with every anxious glance and uncertain touch. The more sincerely you feel these things

YELLOW PANSY
Message: Thinking of You

This pretty flower has a rich history of conveying messages—from innocent flirtation to daring desire—during more *covert* courtships. The joyful yellow variety, however, is far from scandalous. A symbol of loving thoughts and happy memories, pansies are an ideal gift in the early days of a relationship or for celebrating the friendship that started it all. Yellow pansies tinged with a pale purple might even offer a message of hope for passionate embraces to come.

early on, the easier it will be to recall these feelings in trying times.

If yours is a long-established connection, think back to your first encounters and attempt to remember the flutter you felt upon hearing your partner's voice. Embrace the joy you feel at their laughter, and the hot flush of your cheeks when your partner looks at you with hunger in their eyes. And, silly though it may seem, let yourself be entirely carried away with the dizzying feelings of infatuation. That heightened sensitivity will surely follow you into the bedroom, where your partner's very touch will send an electric current through your eager body.

SMALL APPRECIATION

One is never so observant as at the beginning of an especially worthy courtship. And in that time, it is most often the least provocative qualities that we find most enticing. The arch of an eyebrow, that Cheshire-cat grin, the fullness of a lip— everything about your partner seems to send chills through you (not to mention, inspire some delightfully spine-tingling dreams). Learning to harness that spark is as simple as looking at your partner with the eye of an artist stirred by their work.

Whenever you find yourself in need of a lascivious pick-me-up, bring your thoughts to your partner. Look at them with the all-consuming attention of Benedict sketching a particularly striking subject. Outline them in your mind (or even on paper, if you should prefer), paying close attention to the subtle expressions and personal eccentricities that bring a smile to your face. Perhaps better yet, note the things that make you tug ever so gently on your bottom lip. Once your carriage wheels are working furiously, let your partner know which of their finer attributes got them spinning. A little confidence can go a long way in the bedroom!

EMBRACING CREATIVE PURSUITS

When it is the second Bridgerton brother's turn to take a wife, one can only imagine him wooing the lady with a gorgeous charcoal portrait of her. (Between that crooked smile and those talented hands, any woman Benedict set his cap at would likely swoon!) Of course, you do not need his particular artistic talents to inspire fiery affection. If, like Eloise, words are your preferred medium, you could write a love letter that rivals Simon's enthralling speeches.

Do not be fearful of giving your partner suggestions as to how they may put their own creative talents to use. If it would delight you to hear your love sing you an aria, then that is a fine request. And if you prefer a licentious account of your partner's desires (or even a racy bit of embroidery) to a written declaration of love, do let them know. No matter who is on the receiving end of a heartfelt gift, both partners benefit from the surge of serotonin it elicits.

A REWARDING VIRTUE

Although many virtues are prized among the residents of Grosvenor Square, patience seems to be the most arduous to apply. With such a short social season, it is no wonder that marriage-minded misses feel the pressure to settle down. But you cannot deny that the stringent rules that vex our favorite couples in *Bridgerton* made for even steamier encounters. When it comes to building sexual tension, there are few things more effective than being forbidden to touch.

Fall in line with high society's rules for propriety and watch your temperature rise. Start by spending the day apart. Then meet in a crowded place—any of the many balls to which you are surely invited will do—and watch your partner from across the room. Think about how it would feel to steal them away in that moment and head to a deserted corner of the host's castle. When you're together with others, ensure that the two of you never touch, except perhaps to dance with a respectable distance between you. By the end of the evening, you will be racing for the closest four-poster!

ON THE DANCE FLOOR

Even with the wine flowing, the closest any couple can come to truly being together at those lavish London parties is on the dance floor. Share any more than two dances, though, and you are sure to feel the eyes of the entire *ton* upon you (not to mention a sharp reproach in Lady Whistledown's scandal sheet the next day). Whether you attend a friend's nuptials or a charity event, you may still discover opportunities today to don your best attire and hold your partner in your arms. When you do, try embracing those Regency-era rules.

Relish the touch of your partner's hand on yours, and the fact that it is scandalously unimpeded by the fabric of a glove. Hold each other just close enough to feel the heat between your bodies and the warmth of your partner's breath on your cheek. Throughout the dance, steal moments to stare deeply into your partner's loving eyes. And although you may share more than two dances today, try to spend some songs apart. When you finally allow yourself the freedom to fall into each other's arms, you will be as insatiable as honeymooners with a castle (mostly) to themselves.

Dancing

is a perpendicular

EXPRESSION

of a horizontal desire.

—GEORGE BERNARD SHAW

PROMENADE PROUDLY

Now that you have plenty of practice building the heat between you, that shared spark will be evident to anyone with eyes. That makes the act of promenading all the more divine. Although a long walk together in the fresh air does wonders for one's health, your goal here is not to enjoy the scenery—it is to enjoy each other. (And perhaps to acquire the envious looks of those who have made lesser matches.) You may promenade for the benefit of your suitor, or promenade together to put your perfect match on full display.

RED CARNATION
Message: My Heart Aches for You

Whether you cannot stand to be apart for five minutes or you have been apart far too long, the red carnation's striking bloom will let your love know that you yearn for their company. This is no message of carnal desire. The delicately fringed petals speak to a respectful love and admiration, a longing to be near the one who occupies your every thought. Sending a bouquet of these gentle blossoms in your stead assures your partner of your devotion.

When you do promenade, you will want to put your best slippered foot forward. Don a new dress or cravat, hold your head high, and keep a small distance between you. This space allows you to notice not just how tempting *you* find your partner, but how attractive others find them, as well. Imagine being Simon and seeing how the prince salivates over every flick of Daphne's feathered fan. Knowing you are going home with the prize everyone wishes to claim as their own can be delectably empowering.

THE CLANDESTINE CARESS

The butterflies of new love seem to beat their wings at every light graze of a hand, sending a wave of pleasure through your body (and sometimes even permeating your dreams!). Consider Daphne's reaction to Simon's fingers lingering on her bare skin during a perfectly proper dance. She soon finds herself dreaming of the charming rake seductively slipping the snow-white glove from her hand. That is the true power of a lover's touch—it can transform affection into desire in a mere moment.

Putting this into practice is as simple as running your fingers lightly down your partner's arm at dinner, tickling their palm while you walk, or gently brushing the hair from their face. Add an element of danger to your game by

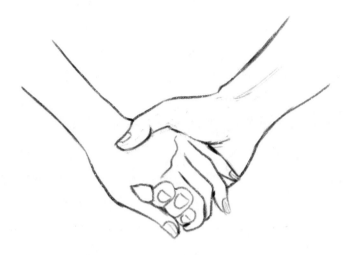

imagining that no one should see you touch. Can you caress your partner's neck or let your hands graze in a crowded room without being caught? Even more intriguing, can you send goose bumps soaring up your lover's arm when no one is looking? Play with various types of touch to discover which makes your partner yearn for your hands on other areas of their body.

AN IMPROPER CONVERSATION

In one brief conversation, Simon provides Daphne with the well-guarded keys to her own sexual kingdom. Should high society hear it, they would be absolutely scandalized. But the *Bridgerton* audience surely hangs on every whispered syllable. Without getting into specifics, whether resorting to coarse language or provoking shame or embarrassment, the well-traveled rake says everything the wide-eyed young lady needs to hear. And his sexy suggestions set a much more sumptuous tone for their marriage. If only every sensitive topic were so easily traversed!

Using this scene as inspiration, challenge yourself to employ the duke's graceful language in describing your desires to your partner. Write things down if you must, but then lean in and whisper your seductive instructions. Because you seek not to act immediately on those instructions but let them slowly burn in your lover's mind, this is best accomplished in a semipublic setting. Let the words simmer throughout the day so that they might boil over when you are alone together.

ALONE TOGETHER AT LAST

Adhere to the rules of high society for even a few days and you will discover your libido recharged and your romantic encounters richer for it. That does not mean you should jump straight into the deep end of that lovely flower-trimmed English pond just yet. Embrace what you have learned and push the bounds of propriety only a little farther (by modern standards, at any rate). In other words, simply let the water come to a boil.

He knew it was the

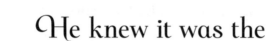

their hands had met,

though she was

perfectly unconscious

of the fact.

—*NORTH AND SOUTH*
BY ELIZABETH GASKELL

When you believe you can take no more teasing, that you cannot live one more minute without your lover's touch, give in to the temptation. Find a secluded area, away from the prying eyes of any society rivals, and give yourselves just one glorious moment of liberty to hold each other close and release some of that mounting desire. Knowing that someone might catch you makes the encounter even more exciting, but it also keeps your time together short. By letting this small amount of steam out of the teapot now, you will ensure an eardrum-shattering whistle later.

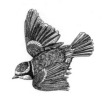

CHAPTER 2

$\int$ETTING THE $\int$CENE

THE ROMANTIC ENTANGLEMENTS involving our favorite Grosvenor Square characters are made all the more enchanting by the dreamy Regency setting that surrounds them. Candy-colored confections, florals spilling over stone structures, velvet jackets and feathered headdresses, women positively dripping in jewels—opulent does not begin to describe the world of *Bridgerton*! In opposition to the propriety of the time, this finery gives every scene a sensuality that takes on a life of its very own.

This, too, offers amorous inspiration worth imitating. The soft, flickering light of candles, for example, is both entrancing and universally flattering. Flower petals blanketing a bed fill the air with sweet fragrance and set a passionate tone for your evening. And do not underestimate the feeling of velvet or silk on bare skin! Whether you prefer debauchery or romance, this rousing section will provide you with all the encouragement you need to bring your sumptuous *Bridgerton* fantasies to life. Choose only the props and techniques that speak to you, or try them all and see which whimsical options send shivers down your spine!

THE GENTLE GLOW

Few things set a lavishly romantic mood as easily (and inexpensively) as candles. Like the duke's dazzling smile, their glow provides just enough gentle light to see by while softening the harsh edges of society. Choosing those scented with soothing essential oils can help you and your partner relax into each other's arms. In addition, candles have a wonderful and underappreciated talent for making anyone kissed by their light look positively radiant. Adding even a few to your dinner table, bedroom, or stone structure can be enough to enhance your evening together.

Proper maintenance and use of candles are a must. Ensure that you do blow them out before nodding off or leaving the room for spontaneous romps elsewhere. For especially precarious situations, there is no shame in using the more modern battery-powered variety. Except, of course, if you intend to incorporate candles into your sensual adventures. In

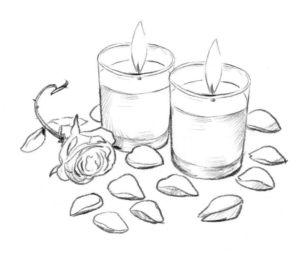

that case, try buying ones used specifically for wax play with a partner. The wax melts into a heavenly massage oil, and at just the right temperature to ensure pleasure instead of pain.

SOFT PETALS AND BLOOMS

Flip through these inspiration-filled pages and you shall find the secret meanings of many common blossoms. In Victorian times, flowers were used to send messages that words could (or should) not convey. A suitor might send apple blossoms to tell a lady he prefers her above all others in the *ton*, and she might return to him a red poppy to let him know that she is not free to be with him. "Conversations" like these must have kept the florist very busy, indeed.

RED PEONY
Message: Bashfulness

These beautiful blooms may be used today to signify romance and passion, but their story is rooted in an ancient myth of modesty. It is said that the nymph Paeonia caught the eye of the famously rakish god Apollo and blushed deeply when noticed by Aphrodite, the goddess of beauty. Out of spite, Aphrodite transformed Paeonia into a red peony. This grand history makes peonies the perfect bouquet for new loves, blushing brides, and fiery flirtations alike.

Although embracing this botanical language may be a fun way for you and your love to communicate, there are many other ways in which you can use those bouquets. You could, of course, simply adorn your home with arrangements of blissful-smelling blooms. But why stop there when you can lead your partner to the bedroom by carpeting the hallway in silken petals? Or drag the blossom of a thornless rose over your lover's bare skin? Between their striking beauty, their romantic fragrance, and their velvety softness, flowers offer endless possibilities for romance.

SENSUAL TOUCHES

With so many visits to the *Modiste*, residents of Mayfair certainly understand the value of good fabric. Corsets are surely uncomfortable, but silk gowns and overstuffed velvet ottomans could easily offset the distress caused by tight laces—especially in the privacy of one's own bedroom. If you should possess such a fine piece of fabric, you might not want to put it to use in steamy situations. Luckily, you may find many alternatives suited to the task.

Drape everyday furniture or bedding in luxurious throw blankets made with plush, silky fibers. If you should want a touch of velvet, wearing a robe made from the supple material—and nothing else—would do just fine. Move your hands slowly and firmly over the fabric to feel the curves of your partner's body beneath it, lingering on the areas they find most pleasurable. When you finally open the robe's ties and slip it from your partner's body, throw it on the bed (or any other available surface) before climbing on top of it. This small indulgence will make you feel like the masters of Clyvedon Castle!

REGENCY FINERY

For the full *Bridgerton* experience, you will surely be wanting even more elegance (and perhaps a bit of royal flair).

Surrounding yourself with luxury—even if it is little more than a façade—can ignite the imagination and make for some very creative entanglements. Not everyone has family diamonds on top of a closetful of other gorgeous gemstone-encrusted jewelry, for example. But an inexpensive replica can still make you feel like a million pounds. Add an ornamented tiara over elegant curls and feign astonishment for an especially apt homage. (And see Part Three, starting on page 187, for more clever ways to use such props.)

Should you not have a three-piece velvet suit available, complete with silk cravat, you may don your best button-down shirt to tease your partner's trembling fingers. Better still, dust off an old tuxedo jacket so they may slip it from your shoulders with a kiss of your neck. With propriety comes layers upon layers of clothes, not to mention the zippers and buttons and ties. Savor the feeling of your fingers on each type of fabric, as well as the time it takes to untie every bow and unclip every cuff link. And, perhaps, leave just a few items in place as your evening progresses.

A VISUAL (AND TANGIBLE) FEAST

You cannot miss the macaron towers, elaborate jellies, and colorful assortments of biscuits around every corner of Grosvenor Square. Part of *Bridgerton* being a feast for the eyes

Life is the

FLOWER

for which

LOVE

is the honey.

—VICTOR HUGO

is the actual feasts featured in every episode. (More than one is the beginning of nighttime jaunts through elegant gardens.) If you are so inclined, you could buy out the local French patisserie and put a variety of lovely pastries, cakes, and confections on display. But there are much finer ways to put food to good use.

A sumptuous trust exercise may be in order here. Use a piece of silk or other soft fabric to blindfold your partner, and fetch a tray of assorted treats. (Your particular state of undress is entirely up to you.) Bring each piece of food to your lover's mouth and let them take a nibble. With their eyes out of commission, they will be able to savor every sweet bite. Let your love enjoy a variety of textures and flavors, from fresh strawberries to lavender macarons and more. Then, when their mouth is full of something especially delicious, deliver a deep kiss. Should you be quite creative, you may find other ways to use the food beyond that.

CONSULT THE *MODISTE*

Daphne may be naive to the importance of a proper nightdress, but Madame Delacroix understands Violet's instructions perfectly well. Eye-catching lingerie can quickly elevate an

PINK CAMELLIA

Message: Longing for You

Camellias come in many splendid shades of pink, but each carries the same missive: missing a distant love. Legend has it that when you send pink camellias to your sweetheart, fairies will deliver them swiftly to your doorstep. But with this blossom's romantic roselike petals, it would be an equally lovely way to tell your partner you long for their touch. Be sure to include a few of these dreamy blooms when setting up for an amorous encounter.

ordinary evening and even make established partners feel like lustful honeymooners again. It is most important to choose styles and fabrics that make the wearer feel good, but that is followed closely by taking your partner's taste into account. However, as evidenced in all the well-endowed women of *Bridgerton*, you can rarely go wrong with a bustier or balconette bra.

Of course, you may also adhere to the Regency-era habit of wearing no undergarment at all. (With so many buttons to unfasten, one need save time wherever possible.) Should you be feeling particularly adventurous, spend an evening out with your partner sans lingerie. Keep the secret until an opportune moment, perhaps during the dessert course. Then lean in and let your love know what you are wearing (or not wearing, as the case may be). Picturing your magnificent body, knowing that it has been all but exposed, and realizing that they may have you soon should be enough to drive your partner wild!

OPEN YOUR BEST BOTTLE

It is no secret that Regency-era Londoners loved to imbibe. Doing so would certainly help stave off some of the anxiety of existing within high society. Consider taking a page from their boozy book and unwinding with a bottle of something luscious. Ratafia would be a fine choice, but any beverage you both enjoy will do. Just be sure not to overindulge or you may have to face some well-intentioned maid's terrible hangover cure!

For best effect, take a moment first to set the mood with a few of the other sensuous suggestions in this section. Light a few scented candles, set out some yummy canapés, and curl up in a luxurious blanket together. Take the time to savor each sip while drinking each other in. If, like our duke and duchess, you are lucky enough to converse easily, simply enjoy each other's company while you pour yourselves a

Passion and

DESIRE

bind your Heart.

Remove the locks.

Become a key,

become a key . . .

—RUMI

second glass. Once you have had just enough to send the tension from your shoulders to other areas of your body, work together to release it entirely.

SLIP INTO SOMETHING COMFORTABLE

Although the audience never sees Simon and his bride soaking in a large clawfoot tub together, we can certainly imagine it was part of their sensual repertoire. In fact, the carefree couple probably spent a fair amount of time exploring many watery possibilities. A warm summer rain may be whimsical, but a hot bath would certainly be more romantic—especially if you add a few sensual touches. You can easily transform a simple bath into an act of intimacy.

When pouring a bath for two, the most important thing is to make sure the temperature suits both parties. (Few things dampen a mood as quickly as slipping sensitive skin into boiling-hot water.) Add a silky bath oil under the running tap, then begin lighting scented candles and placing them around the tub. Their flickering flames should provide the only light in the room. Once the tub is full, scatter vibrant flower petals over the water. Whether you slip into the water opposite your partner to admire them, or you lie together at one end, this is your time to truly relax and enjoy one another.

LET SPARKS FLY

The Vauxhall ball is surely one of the most memorable settings in the entire *Bridgerton* series. Not only does it result in Nigel Berbrooke flat on his back, but it is also the scene of Simon and Daphne's first dance. With an unbelievable array of pyrotechnics behind them, it is no wonder the pair sees stars. (Although, their own electric chemistry could have sent those sparklers skyrocketing!) Arranging your own fireworks display might prove tricky, but there are other ways to recreate their enchanting effect.

Your goal is to capture the magic that Daphne feels at seeing a ceiling of flame-filled lanterns dancing above her.

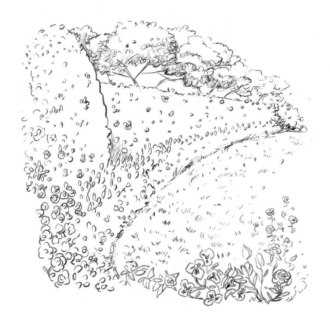

Candles and jewels are a very fine start. But for the kind of explosion you seek to provoke, you will need to think larger. What, for your partner, would be a dream come true? Whether it is watching the world go by from the basket of a hot-air balloon or securing tickets to a real-life ball, find a way to make it happen. The grand gesture is the most crucial part of any Regency romance!

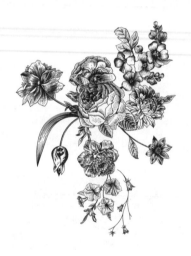

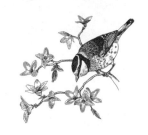

CHAPTER 3

PLEASING ONESELF

AS THE SAYING GOES, you cannot pour from an empty cup. One of the best and most pleasurable ways to ratchet up the level of romance in one's life is to start with oneself. The suggestions in this section (complete with useful charcoal drawings even Benedict would not disparage) will help you do just that. You will come to better understand your own needs and desires and know that putting them first is both natural and healthy. You will also discover how to seduce yourself better than any suitor, tap into your own animal prowess, and share your self-discovery with your love for an even more intimate experience.

Even if you are as knowledgeable as Simon would seem to be, you may learn a thing or two from the pages before you. Having your own pianoforte does not ensure that you know how to play it. And we may all benefit from new sheet music every now and then. Approach this section like Daphne would, with curiosity and an awakening hunger to step into your own sexuality. You have only pleasure to gain from it.

WHAT YOU DO AT NIGHT

During Simon's ever-so-informative conversation with his utterly speechless "friend," he says that the marital act is "a natural extension of what you do at night." A *natural* extension. However improper the topic in polite company, not once does the duke imply that what he discusses is something to cause fear, anxiety, or shame. Indeed, he makes the entire progression sound perfectly divine! What the reformed rake does suggest is that self-pleasure is an integral part of a person's sexual education.

Exploring the bounds of your own body is not just natural, it is *essential*, and not just for its enlightening effects. If you are ever to enjoy a satisfying relationship—full of both the physical and intangible things that bring a couple together— you must first be entirely comfortable with the idea of your body being a conduit for pleasure. So, do as Simon says. Touch yourself. Find what feels good and carry on with that. Experience that release. Once you do, you may allay any lingering embarrassment and fully enjoy your sexuality. There are, after all, better things to come!

KNOW THYSELF

One of our heroine's great insecurities is being completely in the dark regarding the things that occur between a husband and a wife. She instinctively knows that a better understanding could only benefit both her partner and their marriage. Of course, it does help to find a friend in a man who feels no shame in visiting the Dark Walk during a perfectly lovely ball. Simon not only enlightens Daphne—he also draws an effortless connection for her between her own desires and the marital act when he asks her to demonstrate her newfound skills in their shared bed.

Leaning into your longing when you are alone and unfettered by the demands of society can provide you with an understanding of what gives you pleasure and allow you the space to decide the boundaries of your own propriety. And it is the first step in having the kind of romance you truly crave in your partnership. After all, you cannot tell your partner what you want if you do not know. Using the exercise on the next page, empty your mind of expectations and explore your body freely.

Mirror, Mirror

Before you can explore what is in store with your lover, you should know the path to your own pleasure. Whether you are already familiar with your body or you would like to become acquainted in new ways, start by treating yourself with the kind of romance you would hope for from a most desirable partner. Lie down or sit in a chair in front of a full-length mirror so you can see your whole body. Run your fingertips along sensitive areas, from light touches down the length of your sides and gentle flicks of the finger across your nipples, to soft caresses along your forearms or up the length of your thighs. Pay attention to what feels good and let the sensations guide you.

Watch yourself as you go, relishing your own body and paying close attention to how you react with every sensual touch. Open your legs and gently caress your labia—or the outside "lips" of the vulva—and move along the inner edges to heighten your arousal. Keep yourself wanting more by avoiding the clitoris or only allowing yourself light touches to start. Insert a finger or two inside your vagina and feel how your excitement and heart rate change with different strokes: long, slow, in-and-out movements or quick thrusts; wide circles to caress the inside walls; or simultaneous strokes of the clitoris and the inside of your vagina using two hands. Get comfortable watching the different parts of your body at play, and do not be afraid to be untidy. Your body is an adventure to be savored, and it is not just your lover who gets to have all the fun.

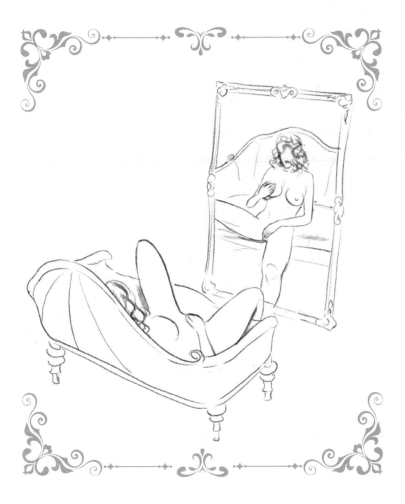

GILDING THE LILY

If you crave romance, take a lesson from entrepreneurial Eloise and cease waiting for a suitor to offer it to you. Setting the scene for your own pleasure is no less important than doing so for a partner. Leaf through the previous section to discover what methods you may employ to delight your senses, relax your body, and find what feels good to you (and no one else). A calming lavender-infused bath, perhaps? Sensuously scented candles? A glass of fine wine?

Make an evening of it! Treat yourself to a delectable dinner, wear something that makes you feel marvelous, and surround yourself with the sensual *accoutrement* that you wish a suitor would use in their efforts to seduce you. Not only will you enjoy yourself more, you will also be letting the Universe know exactly what you expect from your relationship. Of course, if you happen to be in a relationship, it may also help to communicate said expectations to your partner. But doing so will be much easier once you have reclaimed control of your own pleasure.

PARTING THE PETALS

Once you have set the scene for your self-exploration, whether it be a steamy bath or richly decorated bedroom, you need to tend to your emotional environment. Focus solely on physical

DAISY

Message: Purity, Hope, and True Love

One look at the sunny countenance of a daisy and you can see why this cheerful flower offers a message of innocence and hope. Daisies, with their soft, white petals and bright inner disc, technically comprise two separate flowers perfectly blended into one blissful blossom. That is why these happily joined blooms are also said to symbolize true love. Daisies can infuse both your fantasies and your relationship with romantic optimism.

pleasure, and you may have a fine time. But let your mind wander to thoughts of agreeable things (and people), and you will multiply your pleasure many times over. You could think about your partner's charming physique. Or perhaps, like Daphne, you wish to envision the duke's fingers resting lightly on your bare skin. What you imagine is entirely up to you—not even Lady Whistledown will know!

Lascivious or innocent, let the scene play in your mind as you run your hands over your body. Attempt to add vivid details to your fantasy, drawing out the experience so you may savor its delights. Breathe in the warm summer air, or feel the touch of your partner's lips on your collarbone—whatever it is that brings you gratification. As the scintillating scene in your mind comes to its heavenly climax, so too will you.

PLAYING THE PIANOFORTE

Bridgerton does many things masterfully, including transforming the playing of a piano into a sensual experience. Daphne does not just play a lovely song as an expression of her happiness and affection for the duke. Instead, she is inspired by the gradual and exquisite awakening of her own sexuality to create a haunting and complex composition. In that moment, Daphne proves that finding the right notes for one's own fulfillment can be a metamorphic experience.

Performing the "Mirror, Mirror" exercise on page 38 can certainly help you uncover your innate desires. However, as with the pianoforte, nothing but practice will help you fine-tune them. Experiment with a variety of notes and tempos, from the succinct staccato to the lingering legato. Move your fingers from the lowest A to the highest C on the keys. In simpler language, keep tinkering until you are satisfied. Knowing both what brings you closest to the edge of that blissful abyss and what can help you step away from it are equally vital. Consider trying some of the positions in the following pages to help you design your own delicious composition.

The
SEXUAL
EMBRACE

can only be compared

with music and

with prayer.

—MARCUS AURELIUS

Proper Lady

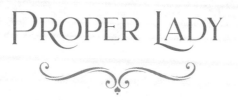

Prop yourself up for an indulgent personal affair. While some women may prefer to ride sidesaddle, here you will straddle a firm pillow to get where you need to go. On a bed or a soft surface, lower yourself onto the pillow, keeping a firm grip on it so you can stay in control of your movements. There is much beauty to this position: with your hips aloft, your legs wrapped tightly around the sides of the pillow, and your most sensitive parts settled against its arch—you will be able to fully indulge yourself while changing up your movements as you please. This position is all about taking action, so do not be shy with satisfying your own needs.

Caress your breasts and body as you softly grind into the pillow. Move in different directions, increasing or decreasing your pace to get just the right rhythm. To feel the most pressure on your clitoris, spread your knees wide and arch your hips back and forth, tightening your butt and pelvic muscles as you go. Do not be afraid to let this position bring out your wild side—allow yourself unbridled movements, whether by arching your back behind you as far as it can go, or by leaning forward to brace the pillow at breakneck speed.

If you want to get there feeling filled, lean parallel to the pillow and slip your fingers or a toy into your vagina by reaching from behind. Tire yourself out as you head toward your climax.

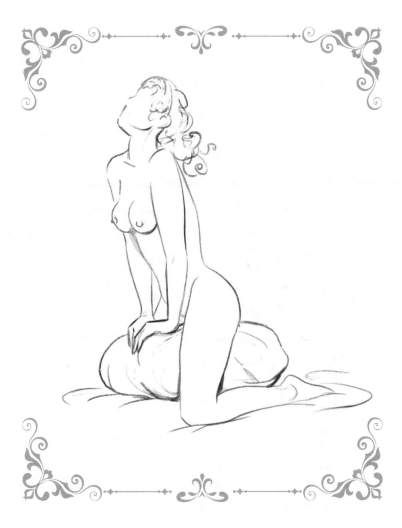

THE LOTUS

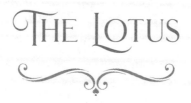

This picture-perfect self-pleasure position will have you blossoming. Sit up straight, propping yourself up against your headboard or by placing the back of your buttocks atop a pillow to help maintain your posture if this helps you to stay comfortable. Keep your legs apart with the soles of your feet touching. To make the most of this moment, you will also need to get into the right frame of mind: Just as the lotus rests gently on the surface of water, your body should remain still as you focus on your breathing and your heightening arousal. Begin by gently massaging your clitoris in a circular motion or with soft flicks. This position is about restraint, which should be familiar to any woman involved in a high-society romance.

Breathe deeply and steadily, keeping your hips still as the intensity slowly builds. The more control and patience you have with your body in its stillness, the more powerful the rise in tension and release. As you come closer to the edge, use your other hand to slip a finger or a small vibrator into your vagina. This position will not allow for deep penetration, so the reward is in the sensual and steady caresses you deliver. Move your finger slowly in and out or place pressure as you circle the walls of your vagina and continue massaging your clitoris. If you are using a vibrator, focus on maintaining composure a bit longer by tightening your pelvic muscles. The control you have with your posture, breathing, and rhythm will bring you to full bloom.

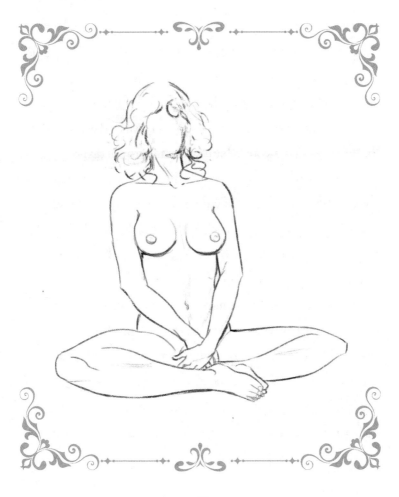

THE SOVEREIGN
THRONE

This may be a hot seat, but here you are in power. Position yourself on a comfortable cushioned chair with legs and place a towel between yourself and the seat. While a fainting couch may seem like a good option for any Regency-era lady, a firm, upright seat will allow you to wrap your feet around the chair legs to make your next moves as controlled and direct as any woman of influence. This self-pleasure position is also good with an audience. If your partner is in the room, have him sit far enough away to observe without interfering. Play with eye contact and see how long you can hold your gazes as you pleasure yourself.

Spread your legs wide and tilt your hips forward so your vulva and part of your clitoris meet the cushion. Move your hips in slow circular or back-and-forth motions so your most sensitive areas receive full pressure from the movement. When you start to feel your heart rate flutter, begin massaging the top part of your clitoris in tandem with your hip movements or with quick, firm taps of your fingertips. Keep your feet wrapped around the legs of the chair to keep the pressure mounting or, if you enjoy toys, release your legs and come down on top of your dildo or vibrator as your orgasm beckons you. Give in to the intensity and use the strength of your hips and legs to rapidly and firmly come into your power.

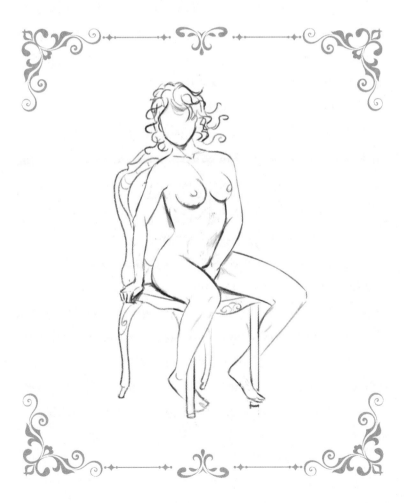

On Two Knees

Even the most seductive of libertines needs time to himself. When solitude summons but sensuality is still near, your gentleman can take up this simple but powerful approach to heightened self-pleasure. He might kneel on a comfortable surface like a cushion or on an ornate four-poster bed. He can sit upright with his heels tucked under his buttocks, parting each side just a bit. His toes and the pads of his feet should be tucked as well so that he can gain strength and momentum as needed. While this setup may not seem elaborate, it puts him in a prime position to heighten his arousal, ultimately increasing the intensity of his orgasm.

As he begins to pleasure himself, he might concentrate on tightening and relaxing the muscles of his pelvic floor. The added focus and rhythm of these Kegel exercises will increase the potency of every stroke, making for greater arousal that promenades him down a path toward an overpowering orgasm. For added stimulation, he should gently tug on his testicles or massage his perineum in tandem with his movements until he brings himself over the edge.

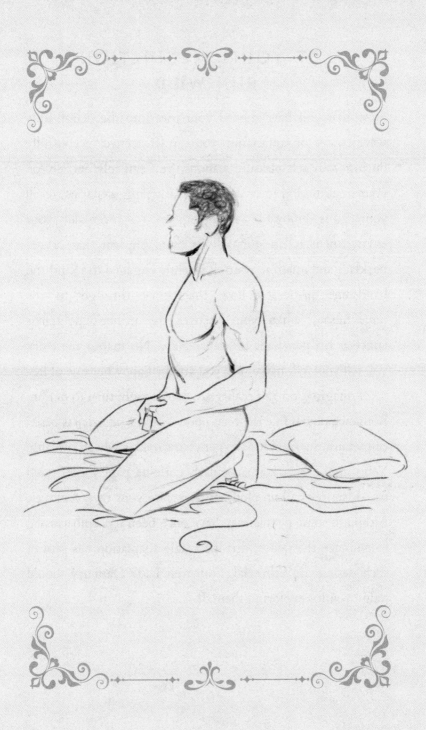

LET YOUR IMAGINATION
RUN WILD

Now that you have dipped your toes into the delightfully warm water of fantasizing, you can let it envelop you fully during your self-pleasure sessions. You can rely entirely on your imagination to create newly satisfying scenarios, recall your most enjoyable entanglements, or even let your environment tell a story all its own. Slip on that crystal necklace and imagine yourself recently engaged to a kind and handsome prince. Follow that story through to the honeymoon, when you discover the prince's politeness conceals his penchant for debauchery. No matter the story you tell yourself, make sure you are the happy heroine of it.

If imagination and reality are not enough, turn to fiction. Romance novels like the ones upon which *Bridgerton* is based can set just the right tone to get your carriage wheels turning. You might earmark a particularly enticing page for repeated use or simply call up plotlines to inspire your own fantasies. Although some people may have once been too embarrassed to embrace the genre, this incredible adaptation has proven such desires are universal. Not even Lady Danbury would judge you for exploring them.

SEX

is as important

as eating or drinking

and we ought to allow

the one appetite to be

SATISFIED

with as little restraint

or false modesty

as the other.

—MARQUIS DE SADE

LIKE ROYALTY

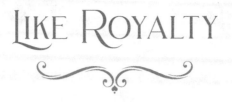

Keeping up appearances in high society can be tiring, which makes this self-pleasure position the leisurely affair you will be longing for all day. Recline against a tower of your most luxurious or comfortable pillows. Lean back so your spine is supported and you can comfortably reach your loveliest parts. This position is ideal for g-spot stimulation because the angle of your back gives you better access to your vagina than you would have lying flat.

As any lady knows, it is best not to rush into things. Warming yourself up with other kinds of arousing touches will help awaken your passion, getting you wetter and allowing better blood flow that will engorge your clitoris and g-spot. As you prime yourself with caresses along your nipples, the inside of your forearms, the creases of your hips, and along the inside of your thighs, you will feel when you are ready to begin giving yourself the royal treatment. Using your fingers or a wand, pulse firmly inside your vaginal wall. Use your free hand to stimulate your clitoris or place pressure on the underside of your vulva to increase the intensity of each sensation. If you are using your fingers, gently create the "come hither" or a circular gesture to stimulate the g-spot. This alone could very well bring you to your bliss, but the combination of active thrusts and clitoral stimulation will make this the kind of orgasm that leaves you flushed and breathless.

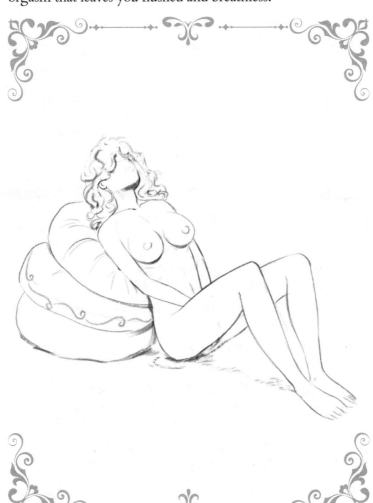

SELF-PLEASURE TOGETHER

One can only hope the exercises and advice presented herein have helped you become more self-possessed in your sexuality. Having a fresh perspective on your innermost desires, you may wish to include your partner in your nighttime (or daytime) explorations. Any suitor worth their spectacular sideburns would delight in watching you give yourself over to your own yearnings. They would also surely be happy to take part in the fun. Self-pleasure can become a most decadent kind of foreplay when enjoyed together.

SWEET PEA

Message: Delicate Pleasures

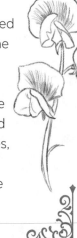

This perfect bloom is a symbol of bliss, kindness, and good tidings. A flower of folded petals that is the picture of femininity, it is the right kind of blossom to tell your partner that he is the one on your mind when cultivating your own budding fantasies. Use these flowers as a token of kindness toward yourself when you indulge your own desires, or share its sweet scent as a gesture of appreciation to your partner when delicate pleasures spring up.

Set the scene for a romantic evening. Light enchanting candles, sip delicious wine, feed each other decadent chocolates. (Despite Eloise's protests, sharing food is an essential part of any partnership.) Then, while staring into each other's eyes, begin to undress yourselves. Act as if you are alone, doing just as you have done before to bring your bliss to its pinnacle. But maintain the presence of mind to enjoy the effect you have on your partner in both body and spirit. Studying each other in this manner will help you provide even greater pleasure when you are joined together.

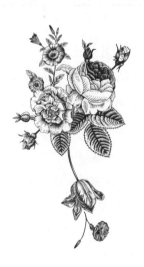

Self-Pleasure Together

Temptation may be at its most agonizing when the object of your affection is just out of reach, but it is also at its most sensual. In this scene, you and your partner are at the mercy of your own desires. Sit closely enough to one another where you can feel the electricity between you—so close you could touch—but be aware that reaching just an inch farther to fulfill those carnal needs would be the very end of your reputations. Instead, you will share your passion by self-pleasuring together. This scene is all about intimacy, not role-playing. Instead of playing to what you think your partner wants to see, treat yourself to what you actually want to feel. You are letting each other in on your most secret of longings and showing them the kinds of touches, strokes, and sweet spots that get your heart racing.

Use your hands the way you would want your partner to—caressing all your most sensitive zones, feeling the heat of your desires by making eye contact, paying close attention to the parts of their body they are most drawn to pleasuring. Heighten your arousal not just by feeling the hot touches of your own hands, but by noticing what turns your partner on most. Talk to each other about what you are feeling and what you like about watching them. Keep pace with each other, and as you come closer to your climaxes, hold eye contact for as long as possible to make this forbidden tryst truly unforgettable.

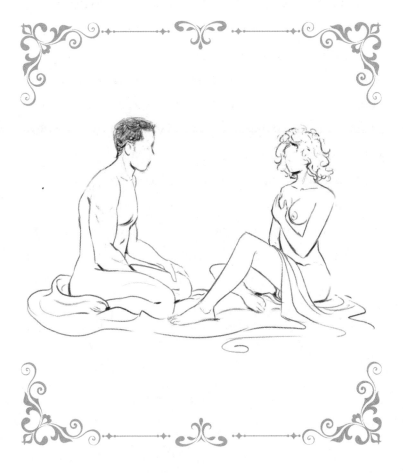

LEARN FROM EACH OTHER

You cannot know what you do not know. Daphne could not have conceived of the true nature of marital relations if given one hundred guesses. Even after Simon's deliciously descriptive lesson in self-pleasure, she still has so much to learn. And her husband is only too happy to oblige. The willingness of the duke and duchess to study each other's desires and learn from each other's experience is what makes their activities so . . . spirited. (That and their palpable chemistry.)

Whether you are as innocent as Daphne or as experienced as Anthony and Siena, being open to learning from and with your partner is essential to enjoying one another. Although no one can understand the peaks and valleys of your body like you do, your partner may yet be able to introduce you to skills and sensations worthy of being added to your repertoire. And you may surprise your partner with your own talents (not to mention the newly formed fantasies you wish to attempt together). Continuing to approach your love with the fresh eyes and curiosity of the duchess herself should keep you both in good stead!

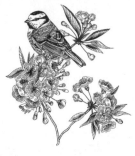

CHAPTER 4

LIGHTING THE FIRE

ALTHOUGH THE DUKE AND DUCHESS often get right to the point in their boisterous activities, there is still much to learn from the way they stoke their shared fire. For it is not just the physical but also the intangible acts of love that lead one's flame to burn bright. Consider Anthony's intensity as he gazes at Siena across a crowded room. Or the way Simon kisses the length of Daphne's neck. There are so many actions both large and small, sweet and scandalous, that can provide inspiration for your foreplay.

Within this chapter, you shall learn how to entice your partner in mind, body, and soul with spine-tingling touch, heartfelt speeches, and heated reunions. Regardless of which suggestion best sparks your interest, it is sure to lead to even greater things. But do not move on too quickly—you may enjoy lighting the spark as much as you do quenching its flame.

DARING DECLARATIONS

Few things can dissolve a person's apprehension as well as an effusive speech (with a hint of sexual tension), and Simon's are simply unparalleled. From his exposition on friendship in front of the queen to his wedding-night declaration of burning desire, he had Daphne—as well as the audience—hanging on his every word. There is no creature on Earth who would not want to hear that they occupy someone's every thought, especially when that someone is a handsome duke with whom you happen to be in love.

Although there are many ways to use one's tongue in romantic activities, the power of words should not be underestimated. If you are not one to make speeches, do not be deterred! A few simple words such as "I love you" or "you look ravishing" may be all you need to communicate your most intimate thoughts and encourage a tender return of affection. As long as you make your partner feel desired (or understood, as Daphne does), you shall do well.

SHARED FANTASIES

Simply knowing that Daphne dreams of Simon is clearly encouragement enough. But we can imagine that, farther down their lovestruck road, they will discuss these things in greater detail. Their adventurous activities would certainly imply a

RED COLUMBINE

Message: Anxiousness and Trembling

Do not mistake this exotic blossom's meaning for one of wearied nerves. The anxiousness and trembling it evokes are symptoms of arousal. With its message of seduction and excitement, a gift of red columbine can tease your partner with the promise of exhilarating things to come. The edible petals also taste as sweet as a lover's kiss, which makes them an alluring addition to a romantic meal as well as to the evening's exploits.

strong appreciation for imaginative sexual endeavors. And the duke seems more than happy to take suggestions from his bride.

Take inspiration from the happy honeymooners and bring your fantasies to bed with you. In fact, why wait until you are already entangled to share your desires when you can tease your partner in advance? When you are in some ordinary public place, preferably earlier in the day, bring your face side by side with theirs and whisper your vision. Between your breath tickling their ear, your lips brushing their skin, and the thought of acting on that fantasy later, you will have their mind and heart racing for the rest of the day.

A GENTLEMAN'S TOUCH

If one thing is certain, it is that there is a time and a place for rough over-the-desk romps, but luxurious foreplay is something to be savored. Allow yourselves lingering touches, intense eye contact, and light kisses to send your excitement buzzing. If the secret to your earthshattering ecstasy is a long lead-in, have your gentleman take his time. Like a daytime promenade where you cannot do too much without causing gossip, have him walk his hands up and down the length of your body.

With the tips of his fingers, he should have the light touch of a duke who is afraid to get too close. His caress should begin in places that will make your heart quicken but only hint at a scandal—the inside of your wrists and up the length of your forearms, the inside of your ankles and up behind a bended knee, the length of your collarbone down to your navel. From here, you can let your cares lighten as he runs his hands down the length of your waist to the inside of your hips. And from the inside of your hips, he can drag his touch

just outside your most intimate areas and down your thigh—
ever avoiding the part of you that will blossom with a more
direct touch. In this scene of gentle arousal, you will feel a
whole-body yearning for him without ever having kissed.
With that heart-racing beginning, the act of letting yourselves
go will be all that much sweeter.

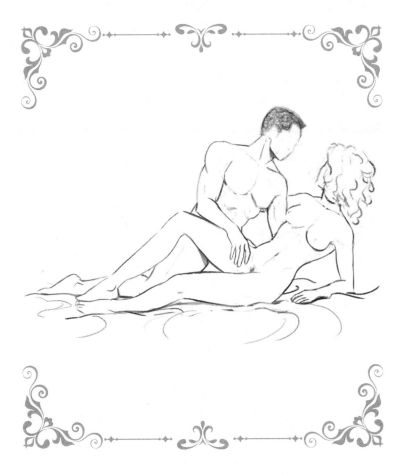

HEAVIER HANDS

As scintillating as a whisper-light touch can be, some moments simply call for a firm hand. You might place that hand on your lover's neck so that your fingers get lost in their lush hair as you kiss them. Perhaps you might sweep your partner into your arms and carry them off to the bedroom. And better still, you might use that steady touch to treat your love to a sensual full-body massage. Few things are more arousing than giving your partner pleasure by running your hands all over their body.

Have your love lie down on the bed. Start by teasing your fingers over their bare skin, then gradually increase the pressure as you move your hands over their back. Grasp your partner's shoulders with your fingers as you use your thumbs to roll over the muscles and release any lingering tension. After a few minutes, begin to explore other areas of their body. Let your hands travel over their arms and legs and everywhere in between, before lowering your lips to their skin. Then slip your hands beneath your partner's body and see if you can encourage them to turn and face you!

EXPLORING EACH OTHER

Although our duchess is evidently a quick study, she may only have an inkling of the full potential her body possesses. The

They forgot

EVERYTHING

the minute they were

TOGETHER

—*WUTHERING HEIGHTS*
BY EMILY BRONTË

duke's lips have certainly been hard at work introducing her to various sensations. But, of course, the phrase "erogenous zones" would be completely foreign to them both. Luckily for you, we have much better information than our innocent (or perhaps not-so-innocent) *Bridgerton* friends.

A steamy massage is the perfect excuse to explore and experiment with your partner's erogenous zones. But do not stop at the use of your hands. Press your lips into the nape of your lover's neck or the small of their back. Drag a silken flower blossom over their inner thigh or navel. Take their nipple into your mouth and run your tongue over it. Use whatever gives your partner pleasure, wherever it gives them pleasure. Established erogenous zones notwithstanding, your partner may take pleasure in any part of their body. Explore each other eagerly to uncover the best methods for you both.

A SECRET CRUSH

Even knowing Penelope's secrets, it is impossible not to wish that she finds happiness with Colin. Her love for him is so pure that, although he constantly looks beyond her, she still works tirelessly to protect him. That level of affection is something to aspire to as well as something that can inspire you. Imagine the delectable dreams Pen must have, and the bold embrace should she find love with her crush! Part fantasy, part possibility, a crush can drum up quite a bit of excitement.

Penelope is fairly terrible at concealing her true feelings, but that is exactly the situation you wish to recreate. Communicate your affection without words: smile, giggle, bat your eyelashes, find reasons to touch your partner's arm. The goal here is to demonstrate innocence but imply a deeper interest. If yours is a new romance, you should have no trouble seeing your partner as swoon worthy. But simply seeing your love through the lens of secret affection should be enough to rekindle any dwindling spark, as well.

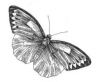

In the Garden

Your love is lush in this garden of desire. On an evening that seems much too busy or far too crowded, find yourself in lust with your partner by creating a secret garden getaway. Start by leaving hints early in the day: flower petals on the pillow, a sketch of a rose on a notepad, or suggestive messages while you are apart. When you cannot stand to be apart any longer, sneak outside and find one another in your own version of a clandestine meeting that could ruin your reputation.

If an actual garden is out of your reach, set the scene together as a moment of hesitation and thrill. Stand before one another, letting your eyes wander across every part of your partner's body: the parting of their lips, the space along their collarbone, the crease that runs down their hip. With the lightest of touches, let the pads of your fingers gently caress your partner's skin, and follow the path of their most sensitive areas. Stroke along their lips, on the inside of their neck, down their forearms, and along their hipline. Let the spark of just-barely touching make your awaited embrace burn all the more hotly.

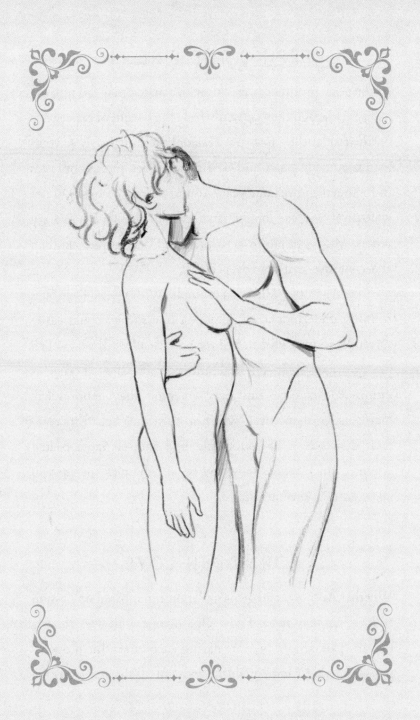

KEEPING THE FIRE LIT

As the years progress, even a true love match may fall into old habits. Although they certainly have the benefit of experience on their side, they may not realize how much they have to gain from trying new and exciting activities. Just as our tastes in food evolve over our years, so too do our desires. Do not wait until you no longer favor certain temptations to try others. Make the effort to surprise and delight one another, and your love will only deepen.

Take Alice and Will as an example. With several little ones running underfoot in their modest home, they could easily surrender to overwhelm. But they are clearly still very much in love, and their physical affection for one another is unmistakable. One can only imagine they must sneak moments for themselves, which in turn may act to increase their desire. Even if you should find yourself quite beaten down, a quick rendezvous may be just the pick-me-up you *and* your relationship require.

FORBIDDEN LOVE

Whether Anthony and Siena's relationship is based on passion or love, we may never know. But anyone with eyes can see that the pair delight in more daring encounters. In an opera-house dressing room, against a tree not all that far from the

WILD ROSE
Message: Pleasure and Pain

Whether its petals are pure white or bright pink, the wild rose is a powerful symbol of love and adoration dating back to the time of Aphrodite. Legend has it that the flower grew from the blood of her lover, Adonis, after his death to honor their eternal love. Its prickly stems suggest the pain of her loss. Use wild roses as a measure of your devotion, or offer them with a sly smirk to suggest that you do not mind a little pain with your pleasure.

road, beneath the bleachers at a prize fight—if there is a chance of being caught, there is a chance of this libidinous duo being caught together. And if you can safely pull off the same, the excitement it instills may become addictive.

Treat your romance as the kind of affair the viscount might pine for, and embrace the buzz of excitement that at any moment you might be exposed. Make uncertainty sensual by embracing the indecorous. Arrange your rendezvous with sly notes or subtle cues, and agree on a location for your tempting tryst. Devise this seduction session in the middle of the day for greater thrill; when other society elites are off climbing social ladders, you will be climbing one another.

COURTING SCANDAL

However charming and kind Prince Friedrich may be, he cannot manufacture a spark where none exists. Daphne's flame can only be lit by one man. The fact that the man is an extraordinarily handsome rake with a hint of darkness about him may act as the tinder. But one must not squander a true love match, however much pressure there may be to live up to the lofty expectations of others. One must be true to oneself (and one's insatiable desire).

Throw caution to the wind and embrace your love openly. Like the lusty couples of *Bridgerton*, let your intrinsic chemistry lead the way, regardless of the eyes of the entire *ton* upon you. Do not be afraid to look like lovesick puppies in public, gazing at each other, caressing each other's skin, and kissing each other deeply. Anyone who might object is simply longing for their own love match, and you are showing them that such a dream is attainable!

The
Act

A Natural Continuation

AFTER ALL THE WAITING, TEASING, TEMPTING, and self-discovery you have dedicated yourself to throughout your courtship (real or feigned), you must be quite ready to be shown *more*. By now, you are surely in search of passionate embraces, wandering kisses, and wild entanglements. This section provides inspiration for these things in spades, allowing your mind and hands to wander in equal measure.

Should you wish to discover how to put your lips to proper use, enjoy spirited activities that would put honeymooners to shame, and give yourself over to your shared pleasure completely, do continue reading. Not only shall you find advice unlike any you have previously seen, you shall also encounter delicious positions in scandalizing detail. Heed the guidance herein and your demonstrable magnetism will be the talk of the *ton*!

Before you proceed, however, consider what the duke himself says: A couple's activities are simply "a natural continuation of what you do at night." You must use the scintillating skills you have gained from the previous section to ensure that your entanglements are as pleasing as your independent undertakings. Approach this section with the same curiosity and wonder as you did the last, and you are sure to enjoy the kind of partnership a certain disillusioned viscount can only dream of—one of passion, romance, respect, and adventure. Like him, you will soon follow in the duke's and duchess's happy and satisfied footsteps.

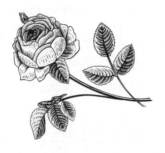

CHAPTER 5

EXPLORING EVERY INCH

AS SIMON DEMONSTRATED on multiple occasions, there is so much more fun to be had between a duke and his duchess than the "marital act" alone provides. Allowing one's lips to travel to other luscious areas of the body, for example, can be quite gratifying for both parties, regardless of who is on the receiving end of their touch. This delicious addition to your activities requires one to submit to one's partner in a way that is unique among all sensual endeavors. (And to see the stately duke submit to his bride in such a way is most satisfying, indeed!)

This chapter offers not just creative inspiration for more enjoyable oral entanglements, but also specific positions with descriptive illustrations for those, like Benedict, who are more visually inclined. You shall discover enlightening advice for both fulfilling a lady's desires and blowing a gentleman's mind (pun entirely intended). Any respectable lesson on lip service would not be complete without inviting one to discover explosive shared experiences, as well. Whether you use these activities as an appetizer, meal, or dessert, you are sure to leave the table feeling satisfied!

BEHIND CLOSED DOORS

In a society that can barely speak of sex without a decree, a deep blush, and several overburdened metaphors, it would be quite out of the question to discuss anything beyond the basic act of procreation. That does not mean, however, that members of the *ton* do not enjoy such sensual extras. It simply suggests that they do not converse about them (outside of White's Gentlemen Club, that is). What happens behind closed doors, however, only the couples involved—and perhaps a few nosy maids—are privileged to know.

Once you are within your own domain, physically or figuratively, what you do is your own business. Explore and experiment to your heart's content! Spend the entire weekend alone together without so much as a cravat around your neck. Submit to each other on every surface in your home. As long as you leave the judgment of society at the door, you will have free rein to discover which positions and maneuvers best suit the two of you.

WITH FERVOR

As in all things, the duke throws himself into his entanglements entirely—in the bedroom, on the lawn, and even halfway up a ladder. When his head is between the duchess's legs, his mind is nowhere else. His sole intention is to bring her as much pleasure with his mouth as he attempts to do with every other facet of his being. This is the kind of passion and focus you must bring to your partner's needs.

Do not move on from oral engagements too quickly. Indeed, let them be the pinnacle of your activities often—your

HONEYSUCKLE
Message: Devoted Affection

This striking climbing vine gets its symbolism from the way it wraps itself around its neighbors, as if it is entangled in a lovers' embrace. But honeysuckle's sugary aroma and bright beauty give it a simpler, secondary meaning: pure happiness. Hummingbirds, butterflies, and honeybees naturally gravitate to this bloom's nectar, which is even sweeter than its scent. Give a bouquet of native honeysuckle to let your partner know that exploring their body tastes equally sweet.

later endeavors will reap the benefits. But that does not mean you should reserve your energy. Although these types of activities often lead one to crave more corporeal entanglements, they should be wholly fulfilling on their own. The goal of any activity between partners should be to bring as much pleasure as possible *in that moment*. The more satisfying each effort is, the more likely it will be to lead to many more like it.

FROM HIS LIPS TO YOURS

With each woman's body responding quite differently to touch, pleasing a lady with one's tongue is not quite as simple as pleasing a gentleman. But it is certainly a most worthwhile endeavor! Knowing that it is your efforts that bring about her delighted moans is its own reward. Of course, it is her enjoyment that is top priority. One thing the ardent lover must be willing to do in the case of oral entanglements is take orders. You may be an esteemed lord in society, but you must be a servant to her pleasure in the bedroom.

Begin with patience, giving the lady pleasure indirectly at first. Kiss and caress her body, working your way to her center. Take your time there too, varying your technique and timing as her enjoyment (hopefully) grows. Each lady has unique needs and desires, so you must look to her for direction.

Listen for the quickness of her breath, take note when she pulls you closer, and of course obey any instructions she may give you. When she is quite enraptured, focus on bringing her to her peak.

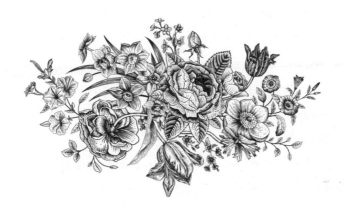

THE ROYAL DINNER

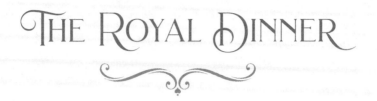

It may be tradition for a duke and duchess to dine across extravagantly long tables, but this regal affair closes that distance right up. In this position, he will treat you like royalty and do all the work. Lie on a relaxing bed or other surface and spread your legs so he has a full presentation of your loveliness in front of him. Allow yourself to become fully tranquil and open to pleasure. Take long and slow breaths, wiggle your fingers and toes, unhunch your shoulders, and settle into your relaxation. Rid your mind of any worries, self-doubt, or pressure of time on the clock, and instead embrace the scene of devotion before you.

Beckon him closer and let him whet his appetite. The clitoris can be fickle—some tongue techniques may be just right on one day and feel uncomfortable the next—but encourage him to taste you fully and help him find a rhythm that meets your needs. He can apply pressure or suction with his tongue as he massages your clitoris, flick gently to bring you closer quickly, or kiss deeply while inserting his fingers rhythmically in and out of your vagina as you approach your climax. Give him gentle cues of where you are by using encouraging language or by running your hands through his hair. By the end of this queenly affair, your hunger for one another may or may not be sated. Feel free to move on to a second course.

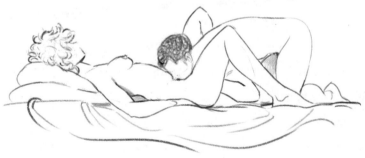

LADY ON TOP

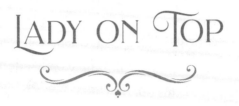

In matters of the heart, it can be unwise to go backward. In matters of the bedroom, it is the perfect direction toward pleasure. Let your leading man rest comfortably on the bed as he awaits your arrival. Slink your way over him on all fours and lower your hips so he can grasp them firmly for shared control of your movements. While this position may seem awkward or uncomfortable, it is the perfect combination of intimate and wildly sexy. Forget any worries about the angle—this is one he is excited to see, and you will be able to tell by how eager he is to devour you.

Let him taste you fully, lowering your hips so your vulva is within reach of his mouth. This is an angle that works in your favor because he can begin his approach with cunnilingus and move back to anilingus if you so desire. As he moves his tongue in rhythmic circles or flicks, he can massage your backside or even bring you to full excitement by fingering you simultaneously. This position is all about your pleasure, so you can remain upright and ride your hips over his mouth as he holds on to you. Luxuriate in the feeling of him using his tongue passionately against you, massaging your own nipples or clitoris to create ecstasy so abundant that it sends you soaring.

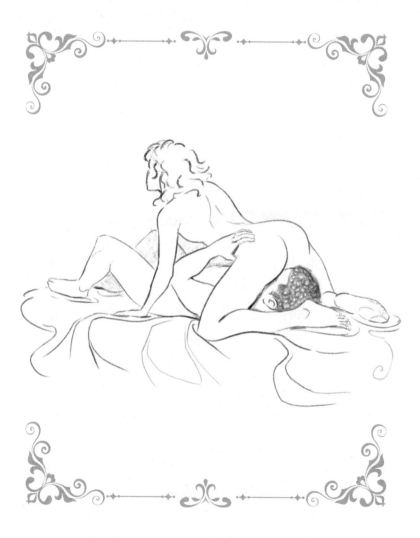

THE STAIRCASE

Never before has a staircase seemed so enticing. When passions are running hot, one way to quell the tension is to let your most carnal of cravings take over. Prepare yourself for an indulgence like no other on a set of stairs or a platform where you can be elevated and he can kneel on the ground. Extend your legs over his shoulders to rest lightly on his back, or spread your legs wide so they fall to the sides and he can wrap his arms beneath them to grasp your hips. In this position, your duty is to let the fire take over. Concern yourself with the heat between you, and let it radiate as he goes down on you.

His attention will be on you and you only, with a ferocious devotion to your eventual release. Here he can use his whole mouth to bring you to erotic heights by kissing your clitoris deeply with both his tongue and lips so you feel massaged wholly. To get you even more wet and primed for climax, he can massage his tongue inside your vagina, run it up your clitoris, and then close his lips for light suction. As your pleasure builds, he should stick with one form of stimulation so as not to interrupt the mounting orgasm, whether that be through intense tongue massaging or suction of your clitoris. Go up this intensely sensual staircase when you want him to go down.

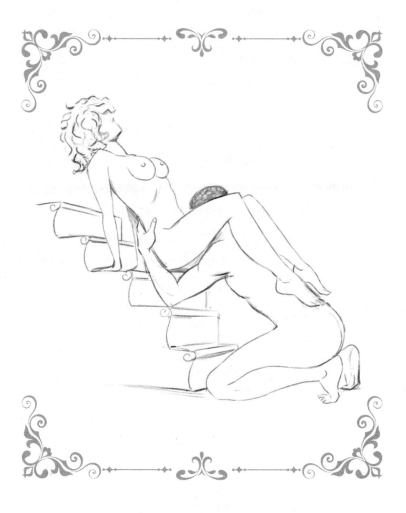

PLEASING HIM

One of the most impressive qualities of the duke and duchess's relationship is that it becomes a true partnership. Each person is respectful, loving, and eager to please their partner. So although we do not see Daphne returning the duke's sensual favors, we can imagine that she did so prolifically. One might be led to believe that a gentleman's needs are more straightforward. But make no mistake—satisfying them requires both knowledge and skill.

Simply focusing your attention on the most obvious area will not do. Variety is the spice of life, as well as the key to any truly exceptional romantic endeavor. Give your attention to the entire area, using your lips, mouth, tongue, and hands to stroke the gentleman quite literally from tip to tail. Vary your movements, pressure, and rhythm often, ensuring that you watch and listen to your partner's reactions. You will know the right time to increase your efforts and bring your lover to his blissful end.

To have her here

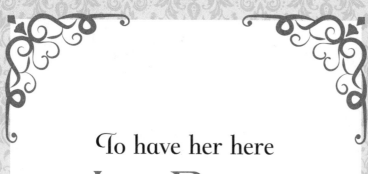
In Bed

with me, breathing on me,

her hair in my mouth—

I count that something of

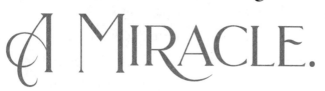
A Miracle.

—HENRY MILLER

THE CROSSROADS

Following the road less traveled may not lead you to a cozy roadside inn, but it will certainly lead him to an idyllic destination. He should lie on a bed with his legs relaxed off the end so his feet hit the floor. On the side of the bed, set up a pillow or a cushion where you can kneel over him from the side. This position is meant to provide a unique deviation from traditional oral sex, with your mouth coming down over his shaft from the side rather than from directly in front of him. The penis is not perfectly round, so this angle will feel different for you, as well. While he relaxes and lets you take control, you will be able to stroke and massage his whole body with much more ease than if you were kneeling before him.

Begin by running your hands up his legs and across his chest to awaken his desire. Bring your hands to his penis and scrotum, gently massaging them to get him going. Lick his shaft and bring your mouth over him, being careful not to drag your teeth. Consider using your hands as an extension of your mouth, moving them in tandem over his penis. This will bring him double the pleasure and limit the need to take him deeper in your throat if that's uncomfortable for you. In moments when you need to come up for air, keep massaging his shaft with a wet hand and rub in circular, up-and-down motions. Here you can even take his testicles in your mouth for a sensual massage that will keep his hunger building. Listen to his cues for what feels good, and take the opportunity to devote yourself fully to his penis and his pleasure.

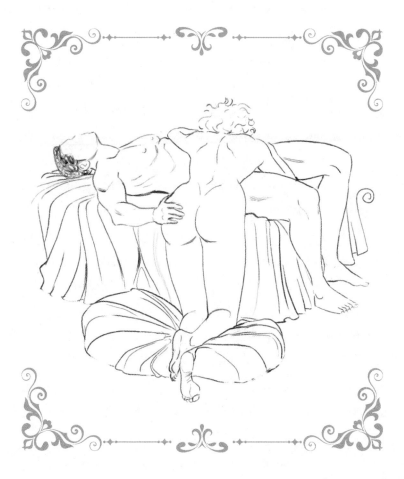

THE CHALICE

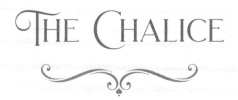

It is his turn to be on top, and your turn to relax and enjoy the spectacle. This position allows him to move his penis in and out of your mouth with gentle precision, while you can focus on exciting him with your hands and tonguing his shaft. Lie back on a bed with your head resting just at its edge. He should stand before you, straddling you so his feet are firmly on the ground but he can smoothly insert himself into your mouth. Hold on to his hips to help guide him in and out, using your tongue to massage his penis. You can move your head to the rhythm of his movements, but do so gingerly to keep your neck from straining.

As he feels the warmth of your mouth around him, you will have free rein to use your hands as you please. Stroke his body with a light touch, or bring one of your hands to tenderly massage his balls or grip the base of his shaft. He may be careful with his movements over you to keep you comfortable, so the extra pressure around his penis will help his mounting pleasure and bring more intensity to the position. This position is so intensely hot for him that all you have to do is caress and encourage his movements as he gets closer to his peak.

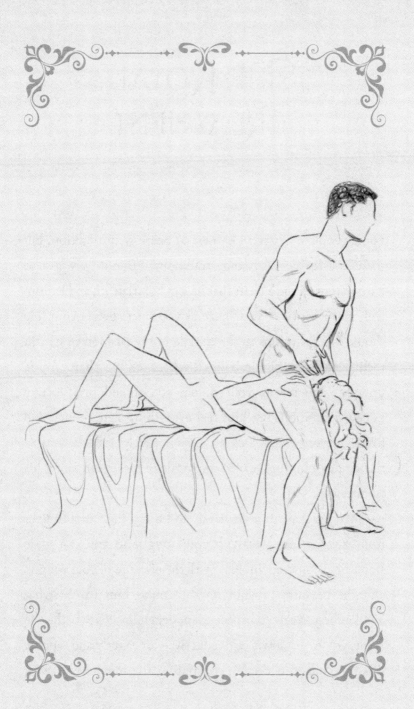

THE ROYAL TREATMENT

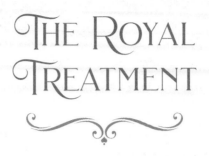

Some people may try in earnest to break with tradition, but there is a reason why some traditional positions are just so hard to resist. Find a chair that he can luxuriate in, and let him feel the intensity of your gaze as you kneel before him. He should bring his hips to the middle of the cushion so he can recline and rest his head on the back of the chair. As he unwinds and awaits your touch, you should find a cozy kneeling position. Let him feel everything here—touch and kiss him everywhere. Lick his nipples, touch his chest, tongue the inside of his hips, caress the inside of his legs or along his favorite areas.

Take his shaft in your hands and bring your mouth over him, getting him wet with your tongue so you can glide smoothly up and down. Play with the pressure of your tongue and the pressure of your hands around him to see what he likes best. Keep your pace even, depending on whether he wants you to go slowly and seductively or eagerly and rapidly. Take moments to rest by continuing the momentum with your hands and watching how the changes in your touch arouse him further. If his body is especially sensitive, continue pleasuring him orally while running your hands lightly up and down his body. There will be less pressure on his penis, but he will feel a whole-body tingling sensation as you guide your mouth around him and your hands along his skin.

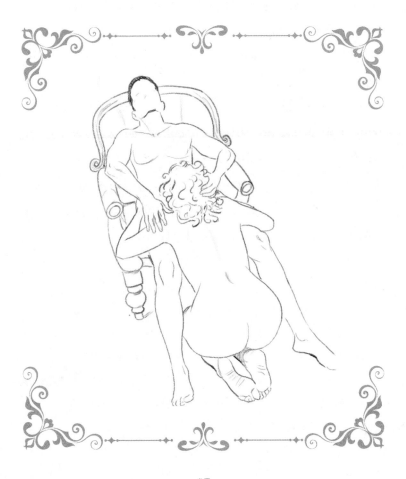

TOGETHER

Certainly, it is admirable and enjoyable to submit to your partner entirely, and they to you. But in addition to taking turns pleasing one another, you can do so simultaneously. Making love to one another this way is as much an act of intimacy as it is an act of pure carnal desire. Every ounce of pleasure you gain you also give. This tension between tenderness and passion makes shared oral entanglements some of the most exciting.

One may become easily distracted in the effort of bringing joy to one's partner, so do try to multitask as best you can. Listen to your lover's moans and let their delight drive your own desire. But do not be so consumed with your own satisfaction that you miss cues regarding your partner's needs. This is a delicate balancing act, at times both literally and figuratively. Use the guidance on the following pages to help you both stay perfectly poised for pleasure.

The sound of a

KISS

is not so loud

as that of a cannon,

but its

ECHO

lasts a great deal

longer.

—OLIVER WENDELL HOLMES

MASSAGE ENVY

The natural continuation of what happens at night may just lead you here. For this lady-on-top take on shared oral pleasure, there is no sense in keeping up propriety and no time to be coy. Reaching heavenly heights can sometimes be a give and take, but here you get to relish in both. Lower yourself onto him so that he can firmly grasp your buttocks, and rest your chest over his torso so you can reach his penis with relative ease. With a little adjustment and very little timidness, you can connect with one another like the gears in a watch. Both of you should form a flow—each roll of your hips aligns with his passionate kiss to your vulva or backside, and your mouth coming down on his shaft will move in sync with his light thrusts.

Use your hands expressively, massaging his shaft while you have him inside your mouth. Continue using your hands, getting them wet with your saliva so they work with your mouth to cover him fully. While it may seem like there is much to think about in the throes of this position, this is one where instinct takes over and you will glide together effortlessly. Let go of any inhibitions, and tap into your darkest desires. If the maids in the hallway are daring to eavesdrop, they will never tell.

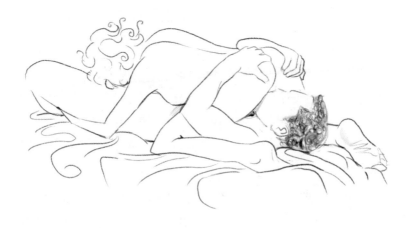

OURS TRULY

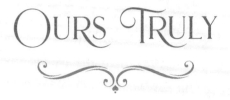

Some furniture is intended for receiving gentleman callers, but atop this piece of furniture, he receives you. Take your tireless lust for one another outside of the bedroom and onto a comfortable ottoman. He lies back with his neck and back supported by the cushion, and you stand over him with your feet on the ground. Your position will give you the opportunity not only to lower yourself gracefully on top of him, but to control the movements—tempting or teasing him by getting closer and pulling away as you wish. You can continue to tease him and draw things out, or you can skip the pleasantries altogether and take him passionately in your hands and mouth.

This position is also perfect for the couple who enjoys the naughtier end of things, giving him easy access to your back end for anal play. Equally, your leverage above him will allow you to indulge him orally with enough room to stroke his perineum and insert a lubricated finger into his anus. Doing so will intensify his pleasure so immensely by massaging the prostate gland that his orgasm will send him reeling. Tap into the more hedonistic ways that rakes claim are theirs alone, and take pleasure in all the liberating feelings of saying yes to your every longing.

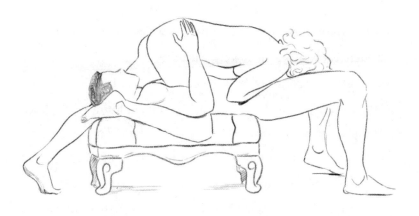

BEDDED BLISS

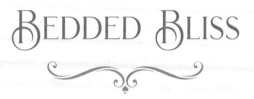

Try something befitting a cozy honeymoon morning. While your energy for one another may be ever-flourishing, there's still time for the slow, the sensual, and the sleepy. This position is perfect for early mornings or lazy afternoons when you cannot help but touch one another, but you both want to keep it leisurely. Move into opposite positions so that you can comfortably rest your head between one another's thighs. Touch each other delicately, running your fingers up and down the length of wherever you can reach. In this scenario, you both should feel a sense of tranquility—doing what's easy and playful without overexerting yourselves. The only cause of breathlessness will be from your budding enjoyment.

Take him in your mouth fully, using your saliva to glide along his shaft. In addition to back-and-forth movements, you can run your tongue firmly along the underside of the head of his penis, or flatten your tongue against his shaft and move it in rhythmic circles. Pay attention to the movement of his hips and the sound of his voice to hear his most vigorous responses, and then make the most of those cues by committing fully. You may have a difficult time concentrating while he devours you; when you need a breath to concentrate on your building pleasure, use your hands to keep him going so his increasing ecstasy does not get interrupted. Focus on keeping your pace even, and the shared pleasure will have you both burning for release.

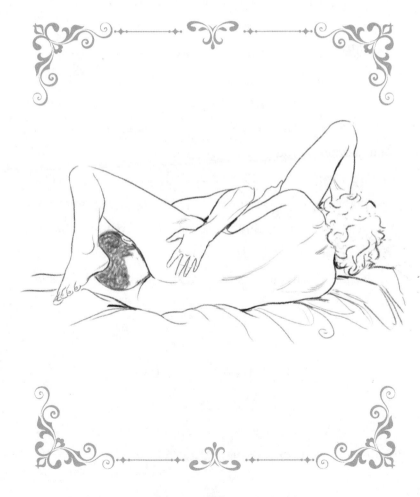

ELEVATED POSITIONS

One honeymoon scene in particular surely had every audience member's imagination whirring with possibilities: the reading-room rendezvous. Daphne's grip on the leather, Simon furiously working beneath her skirts, and that seamless transition all occurring on a library ladder must have launched innumerable fantasies. Luckily for the duke and duchess, their ladder was of the finest craftmanship. Make safety a priority in all your entanglements and you can enjoy similarly spectacular acts.

See if you can carve out some creative spaces for your intimate activities. A secured ladder is certainly an enticing possibility. You could also use a desk or countertop to elevate your partner to the perfect height for easy access. Start by leaning them against the surface and kissing them deeply. Work your lips down their neck and toward their stomach. When you get to their thighs, use your hands to push them up so your partner is on the desk and leaning back. Whether you finish them with your mouth or move on to other enjoyable things will depend on your partner's restraint!

IMMEDIATE NEEDS

When you cannot control your desire for your partner in time to make it to a bed, you can certainly get creative with the location of your activities. A sturdy desk, a nearby set of

RED CAMELLIA
Message: My Heart Is Aflame

One only needs to look at the crimson bloom of a camellia to understand its fierce and fiery significance. But the camellia has an even deeper meaning of true partnership. In Chinese lore, these blossoms represent two lovers embracing. The delicate petals are held together by the deep-green leaves. And, unlike most blooms, both fall together as the flower dies. Bring red camellias into the bedroom to remind you and your partner about the necessary give and take of intimacy.

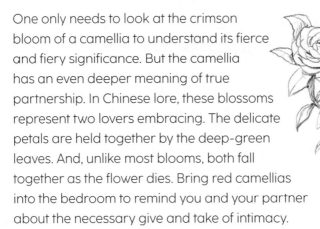

stairs, and a wooden bolster beneath a set of bleachers may suddenly look quite good when you crave your partner's immediate touch. Within the bounds of reason (and with at least some propriety), you too can enjoy such sensuous liberty.

When the moment feels right, search for the nearest space that will compound your pleasure. A private patch of grass warmed by the summer sun, a steamy shower, or an overstuffed couch would all make lovely choices. Simply ensure your chosen surface is stable, comfortable, and not in plain view of unsuspecting spectators. After all, you can only truly enjoy yourself when you feel secure in both your partner *and* your surroundings. (One must be glad that the duke spirits Daphne away to the garden rather than sweeping their supper off that very long table and taking her there in front of the household staff!)

WANTING MORE

Whether you use your mouth to bring your partner to the brink before moving on to other lovely entanglements or you make a meal of their desire for your lips between their legs is for the two of you to decide. And the decision may prove different every time. Some may be happily exhausted by their partner's southward skills. For Daphne, oral activities would seem to make her long for Simon's body. Know that there is nothing wrong with either inclination.

Should you choose to transition to more corporeal activities, understand that everyone's needs are different. Some long for their lover's kiss directly, while others would prefer their lips make a few scenic stops along the way. Some favor finishing twice (or more), and others simply wish to skirt the edge of their pleasure before diving over it with their partner. It will be up to you to communicate your cravings to your companion. Be as direct as Daphne, and you shall have no problem getting what you need.

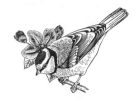

CHAPTER 6

IN THE THROES

ALL THE POLITE COURTING, burning attraction, and lovelorn torment has led to this chapter in our duke and duchess's story. Cue the salacious montage that moves the *Bridgerton* audience to the edge of their seats! The culmination of our favorite couple's desires in a honeymoon that puts Anthony and Siena's exploits to shame can be just as inspiring for us as it is satisfying for them. One need only look closely (and who among us has not?).

From the passionate embraces they share to the way they make full use of Clyvedon Castle's impressive acreage, there are many lessons to take from their most gratifying entanglements. You shall learn within these pages how to read your partner's every shuddering breath, give yourself over to them completely, and take charge of your pleasure. You shall also learn how to make your entanglements last (a lesson Simon himself would certainly do well to study). By the end of this section, you shall enjoy the sort of spirited activities you have been dreaming of since your first glimpse of Grosvenor Square.

HONEYMOONING

Whether your love is just beginning to blossom or its roots are well established, you can take a lesson from our boisterous newlyweds. Enjoy one another! Being intimate with one's partner is a privilege to be met with excitement, desire, and appreciation. You must do whatever is necessary to keep the bloom on the rose.

RED TULIPS

Message: Eternal Love and Passion

As Violet Bridgerton delights in telling her beleaguered eldest son, red tulips symbolize the kind of passion that comes from making a true love match. It is said that they sprang up from the spilled blood of two star-crossed lovers whose lives ended in tragedy, but whose love lived on. Infuse your own romance with ardor by giving a bright bouquet to your partner or even using the edible petals in creative ways.

Try to outdo the honeymooners for just one day. Greet the morning with a sensual exploration of your partner's body. Spend the afternoon together with sunshine on your bare skin. Jettison supper because your hunger for one another is insatiable. And do get creative in not only your positions but also your locations. Treat your love like it is new, and it always will be.

BURN FOR EACH OTHER

Should hearing our duke and duchess proclaim their burning desire to be with one another set your own body aflame, trust that you are not alone. More seductive words have hardly been spoken. And we can easily see they refer to more than the fiery chemistry our main characters share. Burning for your partner means being concerned first with their happiness, their yearnings, and their pleasure.

When both partners take this approach to romance, both are equally sated but also more fulfilled than if each looked out for their own enjoyment. You must not only consider what will please your partner but also show your appreciation for your partner's efforts. Do keep in mind the duke's own rule, though: a gentleman never finishes first. If you must spend an extended amount of time fueling your lady's flame, ensure she is fully satisfied.

DESKTOP TRYST

Getting work done takes new meaning with this immodest romp. Whether you are feeling mischievous in the middle of your workday or you need a way to release stress after a long afternoon of reviewing important ledgers, clear the desk of all your papers and all your worries. Hop on top of the desk and spread your legs for him to have you within his reach. He can start by warming you up, rubbing your clitoris, kneeling on the floor for a few beats to use his tongue on you, or slipping his fingers inside you so this lust in a rush goes smoothly. There is no sense in being polite here—this position is the very pinnacle of impropriety—and you should act accordingly and with abandon.

Pull him inside you with the strength of your legs wrapped around him, and then let him take the lead. You can lean back on the desktop so he shall have a full view of your breasts as he thrusts forcefully. This is also the perfect angle to touch yourself while he drives into you, which will build your pleasure more quickly and also give him a show. If you prefer for him to do the work, hold on to his forearms to keep steady, digging your fingernails in if shouting loudly would cause a fuss. If this is one rendezvous that lasts longer than you expect of a certain duke, have him flip you over so you are leaning over the desk and he takes you from behind. Clutch whatever papers are available to you as his brute force brings you both to your climax.

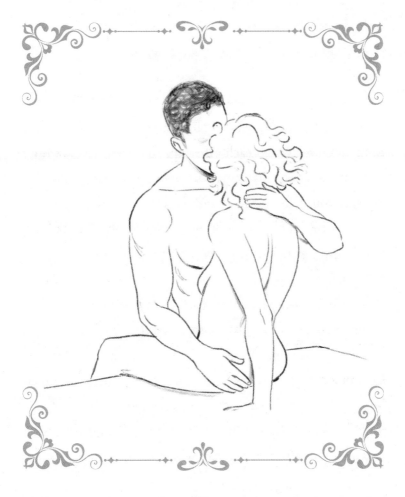

SWEET SEDUCTION

Let the sweeter sides of your passion spring forth with this intimate position. Beckon each other close, savoring all of the little details that fill you with affection and intrigue. Look deeply into one another's eyes, sprinkle each other with light caresses, and stay on your sides for a relaxing entry to tenderness. With one leg over his hip and the other leg intertwined with his, you shall find yourselves locked in a tight embrace. Warm each other up, and when you are fully wet, let the tip of his penis part your labia ever so slightly. Squeeze your muscles so you tighten around his tip, but do not let him enter fully just yet. Kiss each other deeply while pulsing your vaginal muscles, which will have you both fluttering.

When the tension is too much, move your hips forward so he can slide into you dutifully. Hold on to one another to maintain slow and steady control—moving in and out with agonizing discipline so you can feel your thudding excitement. Continue using your muscles to increase your pleasure—he will be able to feel your movements around his shaft and this will heighten his own. The intensity of this feeling will prime you for an orgasm that will have you both quaking in ecstasy.

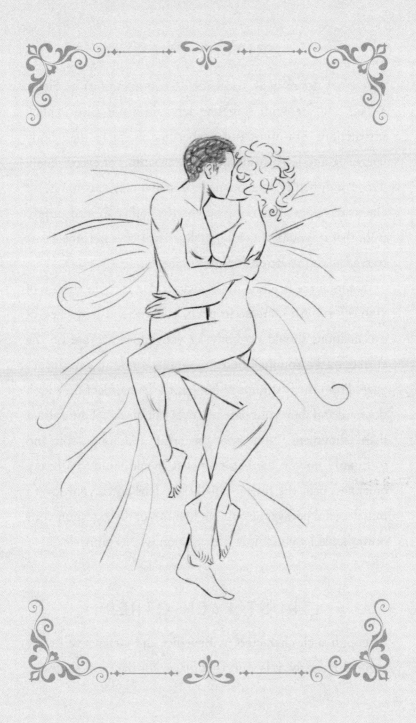

SUBTLE CUES

Not every lover is as vocal (or as commanding) as Siena. When you are with someone who does not give explicit instructions, you must instead become fluent in their body language and learn to decipher the meaning of every moan. This is a difficulty even a true love match may encounter, for chemistry alone does not give you the ability to read minds. (Oh, that it would!) Luckily, such sensual cues become easier to read as your relationship grows deeper.

Sound is the first and most obvious clue as to the success of your efforts. An increase in pitch, volume, and frequency of exclamations should certainly let you know you are on the correct track. You shall find a more subtle hint in your lover's gaze. From the first glint of hunger to the moment they look skyward and shut, your partner's eyes can speak volumes about their enjoyment. Note, too, the breath. Although soft and tortuously slow at the beginning, it should build to a heavy quickness near the finish. Finally, the tensing of your lover's muscles (and perhaps also the tightening of their grip on your skin) should let you know their passion is at its pinnacle.

TRUST EACH OTHER

Although such characters as Benedict and Genevieve might argue differently, it is trust that makes for the most explosive

You pierce my

SOUL.

I am half agony,

half hope.

—*PERSUASION* BY JANE AUSTEN

partnerships. Daphne trusts Simon completely (naively, perhaps, at first), as he does her. This is never more evident than on their wedding night, when the duke asks his duchess if he may show her *more*. Without any idea of what is to come, she gives him free rein with her body. It is this trust and vulnerability that lets the fated pair explore and enjoy each other completely.

You do not need to know every facet of your lover's life in order to give them your trust. Trust, like love, is a choice. Once you choose to trust your partner, give yourself over to them completely. Let go of any self-conscious thoughts and you remain open to the possibility of even greater pleasure.

SWEET WILLIAM
Message: Gallantry and Masculinity

Sweet William is said to be named after the Duke of Cumberland, William Augustus, who led the British forces against the Jacobites just a few decades before our dear Bridgertons make their debuts. Symbolizing the gallantry and masculinity of a soldier, this lovely cluster of fringed blooms creates the perfect opportunity to turn tradition on its head. A lady might offer a bouquet to her own duke in appreciation for his generosity and virility.

Do not hold back, either, in the pleasure you give. Only by trusting your partner, and allowing them to trust you, can you truly give your all to the endeavor. And you must admit, it is an endeavor worthy of your best effort!

MAKING IT LAST

Aside from his stubbornness, Simon has very few faults (that the *Bridgerton* audience is privy to, at least). One of these is certainly that his brevity extends to the bedroom. Luckily for him, his duchess does not know better. But we do, do we not, dear reader? We also know this is an easily remedied issue, with a variety of solutions both gratifying and salacious.

One thing the duke might try during his nighttime activities *sans* duchess is stop at his pinnacle. Bringing himself back from the brink repeatedly by relaxing each time he gets close can train his body to hold on longer. During entanglements with Daphne, he might try switching positions, which requires just enough of a pause to slow him down. Moving your bodies in new ways may also involve a beneficial amount of concentration, as does deep breathing. Finally, he can let Daphne be on top and set the tempo of their activities. Should Simon take this advice, Daphne would certainly be pleasantly surprised by his newfound stamina!

LADIES FIRST

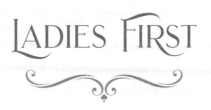

Take the lead, but let it be lovely. There is a time to show your love, and now is that time. A sensual position that lets you feel every inch of one another's bodies, you shall now show your affection with the touch of your skin. Lower yourself onto him, surrounding his shaft, and lay your body softly so you are skin to skin. Pay close attention to how the contact of your skin feels, letting your nipples caress his chest and your hair brush his neck and shoulders. Kiss him gently along his neck, his collarbone, and his earlobes, and feel him firm up even more inside you.

Brace him and move along his length. Keep your torso close and your hips closer so your clitoris rubs against his pubic bone as you proceed. Continue kissing him, cupping his face for greater gentleness and stealing sweet glances to read one another's expressions. If you prefer to keep it slow, engage your muscles around his shaft to intensify the experience, or increase your pace steadily to find a tempo you both yearn for. Resist the urge to come up on your knees and keep your chest close to his, rolling your hips for a stronger grip on his penis. When you both feel close to your release, wrap your arms under his so you can use his shoulders to pull yourself up and down him with more force until you both hit your pinnacle.

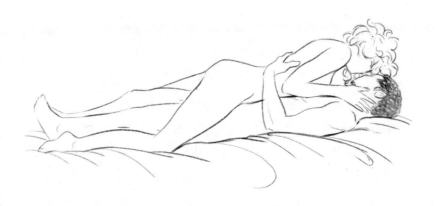

THE SILVER SPOON

A spoonful of sensuality makes everything right. Find each other in a sexy embrace with this demure from-behind position. Start with him as the big spoon and you tucked inside his hips. This angle gives him the freedom to touch you everywhere, so it behooves you to remain still and relaxed while his hands begin to wander. He can run his fingertips the length of your side, massage your breasts and flick your nipples, or bring his hand around you to rub your clitoris. Resist the urge to turn over to face him, because this one is for you.

When you are warmed up, he can slip his fingers between your legs and inside you to bring you pleasure and to feel your wetness. Allow him to linger if you like, or you can guide his penis inside you with the ease that comes with so much foreplay. Use your hips to lean onto him, tightening and relaxing your vagina around his shaft. Move your hips in tandem, accelerating your pace if you are both reeling from passion, or keeping it soft and slow if the scene you are seeking is more sensual. Enjoy the feeling of his hands journeying all over your body, and let him continue to stimulate your softness so you can come together.

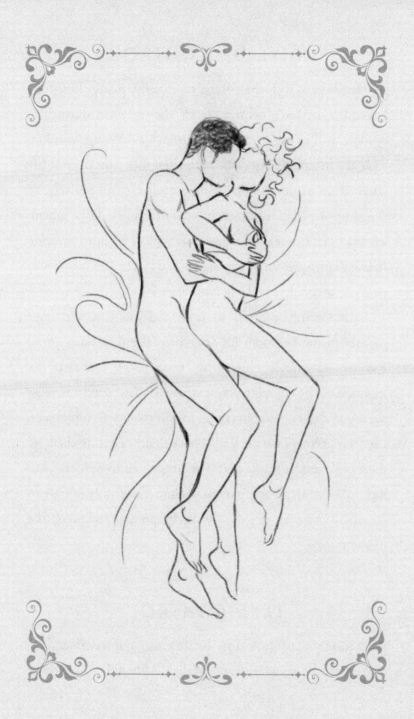

GIVE UP CONTROL

As our duke and duchess learn repeatedly, many things are beyond a person's control, from the weather during an outdoor ball to the unexpected bumps in the long, winding road of a marriage. But some of the best moments in one's life come from a willingness to relinquish control entirely, to throw up one's hands and accept what is. A feigned attachment, for example, can lead to a love that will surely span decades. In ways large and small, the unplanned can be so much better than the meticulously deliberate.

Surrendering yourself to both the moment and your partner in the bedroom (or anywhere else that pleases you) can be an equally liberating experience. Embrace the spontaneous by enjoying your partner whenever and wherever the mood strikes, without trying to control the circumstances. Let your partner take the lead. That can mean letting them set the mood, choose the location, or direct your movements, but it can also mean allowing them to choose a favorite fantasy to act out. Whatever you do, simply be present and enjoy the moment.

TAKE CONTROL

Relinquishing control may be freeing, but commanding control can be a powerful aphrodisiac. Although Simon often initiates the couple's activities, he makes it clear on their wedding night that he will happily submit to Daphne's needs. And we do see her express them on occasion. There is a true give and take in their partnership that allows each one to have control when they want it, and that alone is something to emulate in your own relationship.

When the mood strikes, let your partner know that you shall be calling the shots. You need not bark orders (unless that is something you both enjoy). Simply communicate your desires clearly, and use your body to move your partner's as if you are leading in a dance at the provocative Trowbridge ball. But do note: Consent is an absolute requirement in all matters relating to romantic entanglements, even when handing the reins over to one partner in particular. What Daphne did in that controversial scene was not taking control. It was a violation of her partner's body and trust. Taking control with someone's consent, however, can be a most scintillating experience for both partners.

LEADING LADY

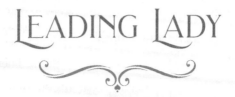

Taking command in the bedroom is a two-person affair. The beauty of riding on top is that your partner gives you the reins to steer his ecstasy, and this kind of submission and trust is liberating and sexy. Do not take a leaf out of a certain duchess's book for matters of trust in this position, but do let yourself lean breathlessly into the passion and strength this position awakens. Start by sitting atop him but not lowering yourself onto his shaft. Bring his penis against you, letting your wetness and labia press against his length without pushing him inside. Slide along him slowly to get him wet and to increase excitement for both of you. Do this a couple of times, making eye contact and gauging his reaction to your warmth.

When you are both primed, slide him inside of you and use the leverage of your knees and hips to control your movements. For a more sensual experience, run your fingertips along his body—his forearms, his chest, his nipples, and even his thighs—to quicken his heart rate. When you are done with being polite, increase your pace to a steady beat. If you are focused on heightening his pleasure, reach your hand behind you and gently massage his scrotum as you go up and down his penis. If you prefer to focus on shared pleasure, hold on tightly to his shoulders or chest to gain momentum and let your hips do the work. Let your body and your desires guide you as you bring one another to the finish.

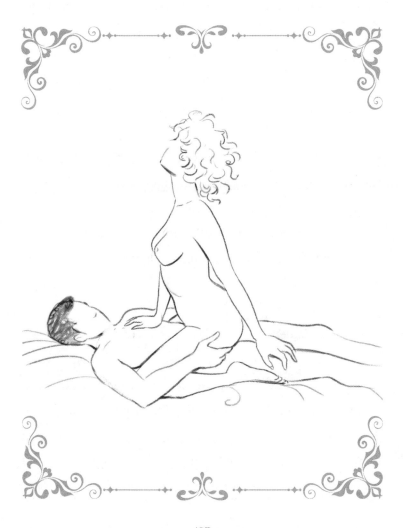

EYE TO EYE

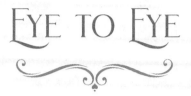

Catching one another's eyes from across a crowded ballroom offers its own special spark, but coming so close that you can see the colorful flecks of their eyes with a catch of the light is something else entirely. Whether your eyes have a little emerald in them, a dark chestnut, or if they are crystalline blue, your partner shall have the time to look over every speck. Come into a lotus position together, wrapping your legs tightly around one another like the vines in a garden. Sit in his lap, resting comfortably in the space between his thighs, and wrap your arms around each other for an even closer embrace.

This position is deeply intimate, allowing you to talk if you like, or focus on the intensity of your connection with your eyes or your lips. Embrace each other closely, feeling the buzz of excitement as your skin touches and as your breath becomes in sync. Scoot yourself deeper into his lap, letting him enter you. You can use your legs against his back to help him move steadily and easily, wrapping your arms under his so you may clasp his shoulders to gain more purchase atop him. As things become more intense, you may find yourself coming up on your knees to gain more control, or even lying back all the way to lose it. But this position is best if you focus on one another's needs slowly and sensually, taking your time to kiss lovingly and profoundly. If you are willing to be vulnerable with your eye contact and your closeness, this position will bring you all the love you are looking for.

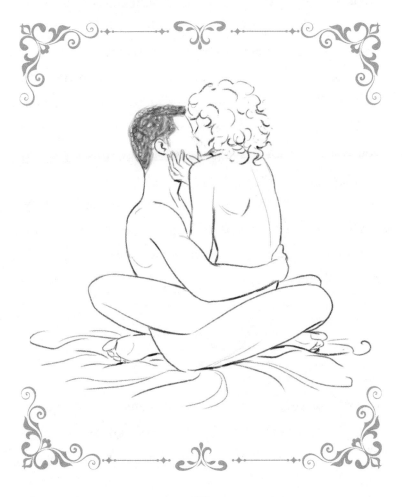

MAKING UP

Although it is heartbreaking to watch Simon and Daphne go through the motions of their wedding day with little more than a self-conscious smile, the confusion does lead to one marvelous wedding night. And when our duke and duchess have the fight to end all fights (and possibly a marriage), they come together again like lascivious magnets. In other words, there is nothing quite like the heated entanglements that ensue after a disagreement—or sometimes in the midst of one!

When next you have an argument with your partner, try using a different tack to defuse your tensions: seduce one another. Like Simon on the stairwell, let your lust overcome you. Whether your activities are tender or frenzied, you may forget why you were fighting in the first place. Of course, if the issue persists beyond your grand finale, do ensure that you deal with it directly. Erotically charged anger may be exciting, but it is only a matter of time before the anger is all that is left. A lovingly resolved dispute, on the other hand, may lead you to honeymoon-esque entanglements!

REIGNITE THE SPARK

In the embraces of new love, it is only natural to have trouble controlling one's passions. You crave your lover's touch, you long to know their every sensual wish, you need to explore their body freely. You are quite open to new experiences because everything is, inherently, a new experience. As you grow older, however, you may fall into a familiar rhythm. Trusted and sufficient as that tempo may be, it is time to compose new, more provocative music together!

Break out of old habits by making a new one; add at least one new experience to each of your entanglements. Begin, perhaps, by adding a new position to your repertoire. (Turn to the next chapter for inspiration on this front.) And do not be tempted to scoff at any you find silly or intimidating. Simply attempting something new will bring that early boldness back to your partnership. Why not court scandal and take your activities beyond the bedroom walls as well? And do not forget to look to your own libidinous past, perhaps even recreating your most explosive entanglements. As Henry Granville would tell you, inspiration is everywhere!

The greatest

PLEASURE

of life is

LOVE.

—EURIPIDES

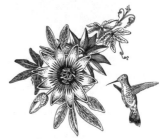

CHAPTER 7

MORE
DELICIOUS
POSITIONS

I DID SAY I WOULD NOT LEAVE YOU in the dark like the tongue-tied mamas of the *ton*, and a lady always keeps her promises. Should you tend more toward Benedict's visual inclinations than Pen's proficiencies in prose, this chapter will be a most cherished companion on your sensual journey. In it you shall find not just salacious instructions for the most exquisitely libidinous positions, but also delectable charcoal sketches that shall help you envision your part completely.

The advice that accompanies these steamy illustrations is far more enlightening than any speech by either the mortified Lady Bridgerton or the seductively effusive Duke of Hastings himself. You shall understand perfectly how to maneuver yourself and your partner into the most sinfully delicious positions and the exact methods for extracting the most pleasure from each. Whether you pick and choose the more intriguing or you set out to try them all, your romantic life shall only be the better for it!

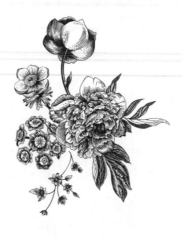

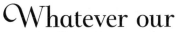

Whatever our

SOULS

are made of,

his and mine

are the same.

—*WUTHERING HEIGHTS*
BY EMILY BRONTË

HELLO, YOUR GRACE

Some greetings are superior to others, and here you shall introduce your partner to your most confident self. Choose a chair without arms so you both have room to move uninhibited. Lower yourself onto him and scoot your hips as close to his as you can so your pubic bones are touching. This will give you more direct clitoral stimulation as you begin to slide up and down his shaft. You will be in the perfect position to focus on kissing each other passionately, taking time to be tender with your touches and offer each other long-lasting eye contact. Let the thrill of your tongues against one another boost the thrill of feeling him inside you, keeping a sensual cadence.

As your excitement begins to climb, use his shoulders or the back of the chair to gain momentum and the strength of your legs on the floor to control your movements. Ride against him as if your pace could stop an ill-fated duel, and allow yourself to be unrestrained in your efforts. Keep your clitoris against his pubic bone as you pick up your speed and come closer to climax. When the time is right you can reach your pinnacle with full g-spot and clitoral stimulation for you, and breathless release for him.

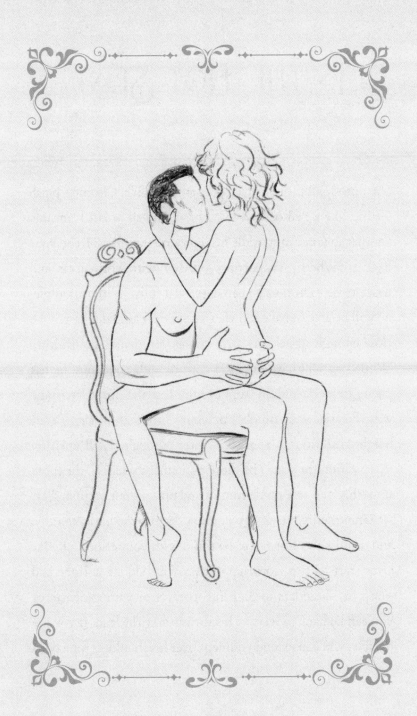

In the Hot Seat

Slip onto something a little more comfortable. Choose a plush setting like a bed or a large cushion, and sit across from one another so you can straddle his hips with your legs. Keep your back straight by supporting yourself with your arms and move close to him so he can enter you fully. With this angle, he will be able to have full view of your breasts, and he will be close enough so he can caress you as you grind against him. While you will have the most control with your hips, he has plenty to work with in front of him. Instruct him to massage your breasts, your nipples, or your clitoris as you go. Your heightened arousal from these intense touches will open up this position for you. The more excitement you feel, the more smoothly you can guide him in and out of your vagina.

Unburden yourself as you go by feeling the pleasure fully, and dismiss any instinct to be timid with your efforts. If your arms start to tire from supporting yourself, sit upright and grasp his shoulders to gain full control of your cadence, or you can lie back to relax so his thrusts take the lead. If you are flexible, you can extend your legs over his shoulders for a deep penetration that will hit your g-spot and that will surround him completely. This position may not be reserved for polite society, but it will leave you both feeling well bedded.

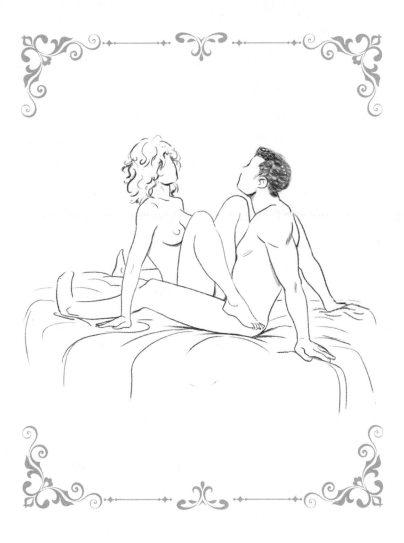

THE RAKE

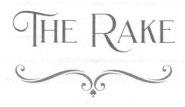

A rake takes what he wants, and in this seductive stance, he will take you to tantalizing heights. Prop your back against a pillow or have him place a firm arm behind you for support. The beauty of this position is multifaceted; the angle of your hips and snugness of your closed thighs create a tighter grip around him that you might not experience facing one another directly or even from behind. While he enjoys a full view of your breasts and firmer, deeper sensations as he moves inside you, the pressure from your closed legs will allow for indirect clitoral stimulation.

Begin slowly, letting him slide smoothly in and out of you with the tender precision of a man who knows patience is the most gratifying of virtues. Massage your own breasts to increase stimulation or let him do so for you. In this role, you get to play coy while he lets his wilder whims get the best of him. While he may have the upper hand in this wanton scene suitable for a rake, you have just as much control with your hip movements and vaginal muscles. Move confidently in tandem with him as you let your passion find its peak.

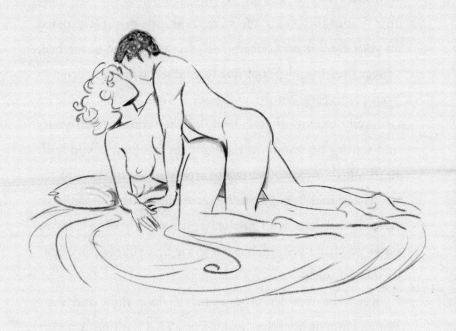

Sweet Nothings

Whispers may be circling within the *ton*, but the only ones that matter to you are the sweet nothings being whispered in your ear. Lie on your stomach facing the end of the bed. Hover over the edge and steady yourself with your arms so your palms press firmly on the floor. Your partner should lie delicately on top of you, bringing his arms around yours and setting his hands on the floor for stability. If you both need a little time to warm up, arch your buttocks into his pelvis and rock together to increase one another's readiness. Spread your legs with just enough room to allow him to enter you from behind, but not so far that your legs are bent or splayed wide.

Keep the muscles of your pelvic floor tight and your bodies close as he moves inside you. This position is meant for closeness, so stay parallel as you move in unison. As you move gingerly together, he will be able to massage your breasts and nipples periodically. If your arms languish from keeping yourselves steady on the floor, move them into a candelabra shape and interlock fingers with your partner for steadiness. Keep your bodies pressed together and move your hips in circles to keep up the sensual momentum.

Enjoy shared whispers that not even the town gossips would dare repeat.

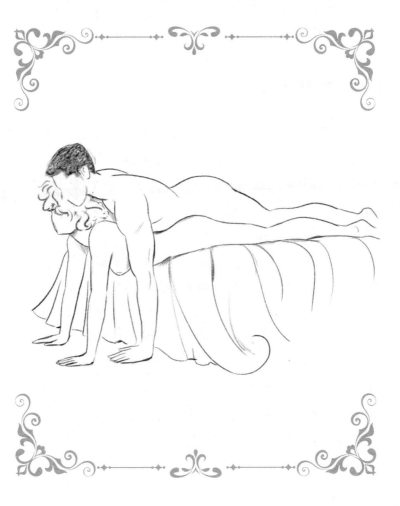

THE DUCHESS

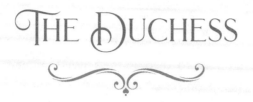

It is time to test all the furnishings in your new countryside castle. In this position, you get full control while he gets to sit back and gain a relaxing view of your backside. Choose a chair without arms or with a wide seat so you can drape your legs on either side of his torso. It is best to move into this position from a reverse-straddle, lowering yourself onto his penis and clicking in like a lock and key. Gingerly move forward to rest your elbows on an ottoman or a cushioned bench to stabilize yourself, being careful to pivot your pelvis to keep him inside you without bending him.

Grasp the edge of the bench so you have a firm grip, but focus on using your hips and knees to slide back and forth along his shaft. Your arms may tire if you rely on a pull-up motion. It helps to be extra wet while getting into the groove of this super-sultry position, so he should spend his leisure time caressing your body, running his fingers along sensitive parts of your feet and up your legs, and getting a good grip on your derriere. While it may be custom for certain Regency couples to only speak through sex, this is one position that can benefit from good communication. Tell each other what feels good, and use enthusiastic language or sounds to check in since you will not be making eye contact. Enjoy the thrill of finding new ways to bring each other to heavenly heights.

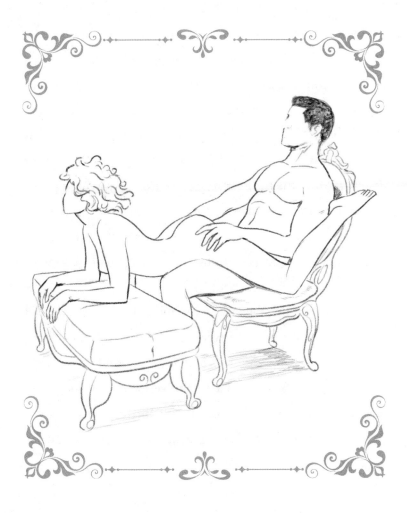

Hold Me Tight

Sometimes you just cannot keep your hands off one another, and a quiet afternoon tea becomes a passionate romp against the nearest surface. This lusty L-shape makes the most of a tight embrace, but this has nothing to do with wrapping your arms around one another. Start in a standing position, allowing him to enter you as if you were going to fulfill your love and lust upright. He should kneel on a seat cushion or couch, finding the right balance so he can tip you back across the edge and wield you as he sees fit. Bring your legs up over his shoulders and squeeze your legs tightly so you hug his penis snugly. For an even tighter fit, cross your legs so your feet rest on his opposite shoulders.

In a position that penetrates you more deeply than a raised eyebrow or seductive stare ever could, he controls the steamy scene by supporting your hips and lower back while carrying you to oblivion. Be sure to have your back and spine supported with a pillow or a soft blanket if your furniture is better for show than for comfort. This angle shall give him a spectacular view of the movement of your breasts as he drives into you, and if he has an especially good grip, he can use a free hand to caress you. Brace against his arms or the arms of the chair as you both come into your most indecorous ecstasy.

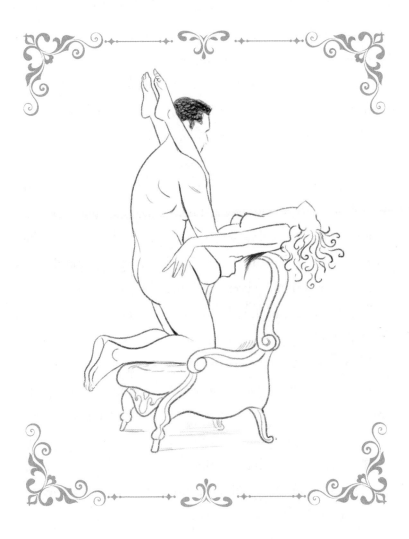

THE CHARIOT

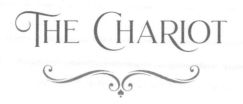

His chariot awaits with this provocative position. After the niceties of a civilized courtship, it is no wonder the walls of modesty fall away. Take him to alluring heights by beckoning him inside your chariot. It goes without saying that this position requires you both to be primed and ready, so be sure to spend the time to tempt, tease, and tantalize each other before jumping in. Find a stable surface, like a table, bed, or anything with sturdy legs at knee or waist height that will support you. Lean down and place your palms against the surface with your backside facing him. Ever so gently, he should pick you up by your legs and hold you by your thighs. Tighten your stomach as he does this so you do not wobble, and wrap your feet behind his back to close up the position.

From here, he is the driver. Get ready for deep penetration that he can deliver with a sensual, steady pace, or in quick movements that will have you clawing at the table. Use your hips and feet to move in tandem with his thrusts for a strong and united flow. No one said a gentleman has to be gentle, so let this position be your awakening to a more powerful destination. Be vocal with your needs and level of excitement—

if this angle is too intense, let him know to moderate how deep he goes. If it is exactly what you need, encourage him to drive you home.

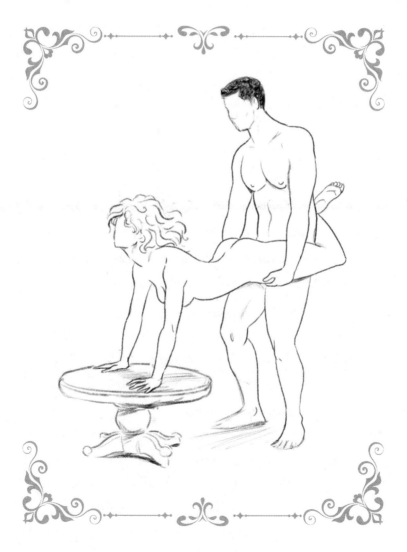

SUMMER BLOSSOM

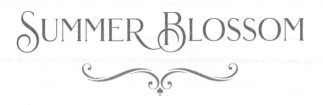

No love story is complete without the perfect bouquet of flowers, so let your love come to full bloom with this pretty arrangement. Let him lie back while he is fully aroused. Place yourself facing away from him in a cross-legged position, bringing him snugly inside you when you are well lubricated. Be sure to rest your ankles on his thighs so your position is secure, avoiding any pressure on sensitive areas like his knees. Because this flowering stance is so delicate, the emphasis will be on slow gyrations, strong muscle tightening, and sensual touching. Taking this to wilder gardens will require you to bring your knees down onto the bed for better control so you do not hurt his legs or your ankles.

Focus on tender touches, running your fingertips along his sensitive areas and even touching yourself so he knows you are excited. Tighten and loosen your pelvic floor muscles in a constant rhythm, building pressure on his penis and intensifying your gradual climb toward climax. You will have ready access to his scrotum, so play by massaging and gently tugging for good measure. Lick your middle finger and move it along his perineum and into his backside if this pleases him. Gently massage in tandem with the tightening of your vaginal muscles so his pleasure builds as quickly as yours. If he is not too overwhelmed, he can sit up to embrace you and massage your clitoris from behind. If he is, you can touch yourself with one hand and send his bliss soaring with the other.

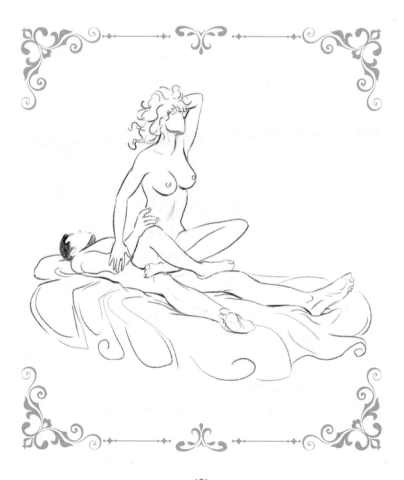

THE NEWLYWEDS

Flip the standards of high society as you get flipped over on your promenade for pleasure. This position has no limit to its opportunity—find yourselves in bedded bliss in silken sheets on a cozy morning, turn a countryside picnic into a leisurely love affair, or slink into sensuality on any cushioned surface. The feeling of each other's skin will be what sends this position sailing, so begin with soft kisses and gentle touching. Run your hands along each other's bodies and build an extra level of tension that you reserve for lazy days when you are feeling desirous, but not ravenous. Touch and kiss each other softly, and when the thudding intensity gets to be too much, flip over to present your backside to him.

Pleasure is just a connection away, and here he can move inside you closely. Keep your bodies near so you can glide sultrily in unison rather than moving onto your knees for more aggressive thrusts. By staying close together and against the surface below, you can tighten yourself around his shaft while also placing pressure on your clitoris. This will help you bring your lust closer to orgasm and will grow his thirst.

Be sure to clutch, grip, or claw at the closest cushion, because you are sure to feel deep stimulation that will leave you breathless.

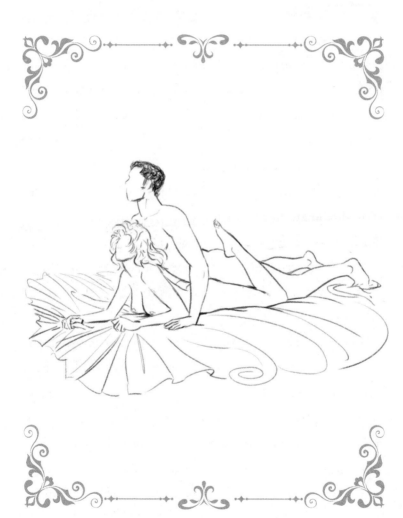

LADY IN WAITING

It may require a lot of pomp and circumstance to attract a gentleman during the social season of the *ton*, but in this position he shall be coming to you. Lie face down on a bed and let him caress you all over, getting you ready for his arrival. Spread your legs so he might pull your thighs to him to rest your hips atop his. Let him generously massage you, rubbing his hands up and down your back, palming your behind, and running a firm thumb from the inside of your knees up to the inside of your thighs where your bodies meet. When he is ready to move inside you, brace your thighs gently so you can circulate your hips to move up and down his shaft.

Let it be known that this stance is yours to enjoy. Sprawl yourself out, letting him stroke you as he lifts his hips back and forth to move inside you. If you are looking for a more rapid pace, he can lift his hips up to a bridge position so he is moving firmly into you, letting you move along with him and his rhythm. If he remains close to the bed and pulls toward you with his feet rather than thrusting up with his hips, gyrate your pelvis in methodical circles to add more heat. Let your clitoris rub against the surface below, feel him move against your most sensitive spots, and clutch the closest bedsheet as you move toward bliss.

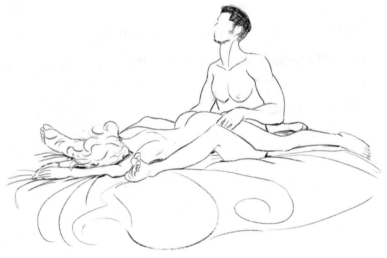

THE MAIDEN VOYAGE

Boating on the Thames has its downfalls, but avoid the scuffle and set your sights on the bow of the ship. Let him lie on a comfortable seat and spread yourself out atop him like the mermaid you were intended to be. Rest your hands just above his knees and have him hold on tightly to your pelvis. You will want to keep your feet firmly on the floor for the majority of this entanglement to keep your balance and to give yourself more leverage as you move. You may begin with a slow pace to get things started, but this is one position that does not stay relaxed for long. As you quicken your pace on top of him, he can use his strength to help bring your hips up and down so that you are sharing the work and you can keep going longer.

If you must catch your breath, move your legs from straddling the outside of his legs to instead sitting between them. This will create a tighter fit around him, and you can relax your pace while you ramp up for more. As you come closer to the brink, return to your original position with your legs at his sides. Have him grasp you by the hips or wrap his arms around your waist. Clutch your knees against his sides to maintain position, and arch your torso up so you can feel the promise of a heavenly arrival.

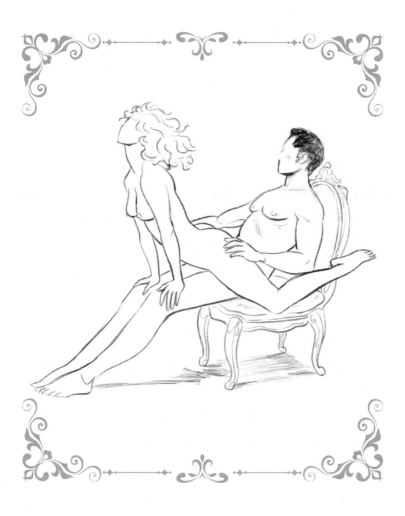

THE ENTANGLEMENT

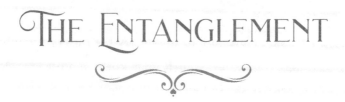

Get entwined in more than just town gossip. In this sensual scenario, you are laid out in the most leisurely of postures, with nothing to concern yourself with but the euphoria that awaits. Enjoy the luxury of having all your needs cared for by the one who knows all your sweet spots. Lie back and let your partner feel his way across your skin, from the inside of your hips and up your side to the sensitive skin of your forearms. Have him caress your breasts, paying special attention to your nipples. With soft kisses and steady flicks to this most libidinous zone, you will feel a warming in your clitoris that—with enough dedication—can bring you all the way to your peak.

Your gentleman should position himself behind you as if he were about to spoon you. Open your legs to accept him into your loveliness between. When he has slid inside, wrap one leg around his to straddle it. Keep your back flat on the bed, and let him work his way in and out of you while you enjoy the bliss. With his free hand or yours, rub your clitoris with gentle pressure to feel multiple avenues of ecstasy.

Speak openly about what you are feeling, sharing what movements spark your fire as you go. Keep the flames burning until you can no longer handle it, and come together in a passionate embrace.

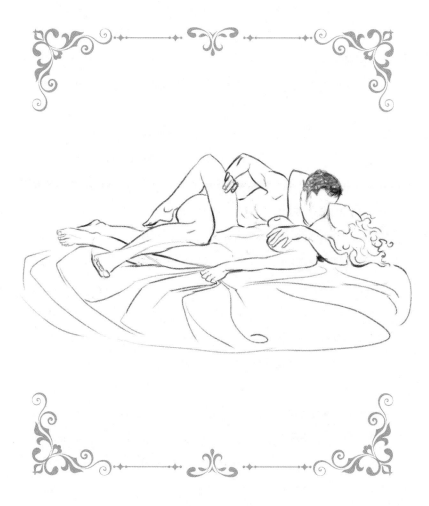

THE DANCER

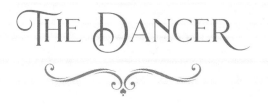

You might twirl your way onto the dance floor like all the rest of the ladies of the *ton*, or you could twirl your way into bed. A position that offers an admiring view of your breasts, it is also generous in its depth. Sprawl onto the bed, drawing him in with your gaze. As he kneels before you with his back as straight as a rod, raise your legs and elegantly land them on his shoulders. He shall take your legs in his arms as he might take you on the dance floor, and he can move gently to enter you. Grasping your hips or backside for good measure, he will have the power to speed up the tempo or slow it down.

With your hips raised at an angle against his knees and your legs closed tightly, he will be able to move deeper inside you than ever before. While this position could allow you to lie back and let these tantalizing moments merely happen to you, you could move your pelvis in unison with his so you are complementing every thrust inside you. Touch him wherever you can reach, including his forearms, thighs, and backside. As you both come closer to the best part of this recital, make long-lasting eye contact that will allow the world to fall away.

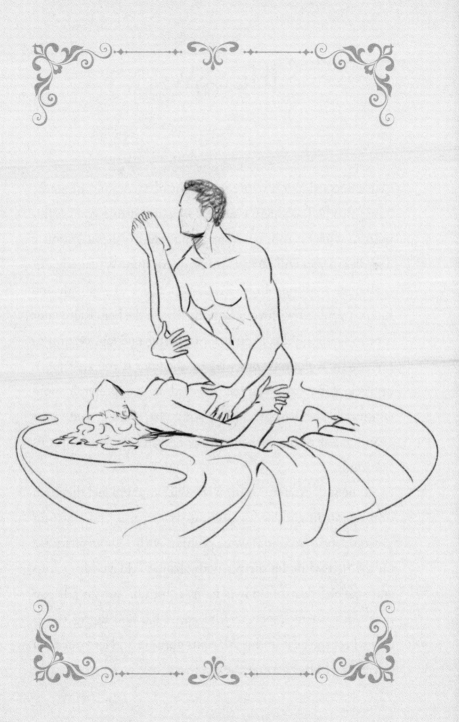

The Swan

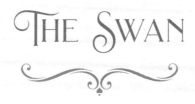

Swim into seduction with this delightful encounter. Begin by lying on a bed or chaise lounge. Have him prime you for this posture with his tongue, giving your clitoris the attention it deserves so you will be wet and ready for him. When you can no longer wait to feel him inside you, move to your side and support yourself with your arms firmly on the bed. Raise your hips to fit snugly between his, extending one leg for him to hold on to. Keep your other leg on the floor if you are supple, or tuck it beneath you on the bed if you prefer a more comfortable extension. With your leg raised and your exquisiteness open, have him drive deep inside you from this side angle.

As he will be coming from the side, you will feel the girth of his penis in a fuller way, filling your vagina and reaching greater depths. Maintain your position with your arms strong on the bed while he thrusts with abandon. Have him caress and squeeze your bottom as he goes, or ask him to tell you how your warmth feels to him and what it is doing to his body. Feel the heat of this salacious position and let your wild side free. If after a time the approach begins to strain your hips or leg, bring yourself down onto the bed and have him glide into you from behind. Stretch out onto your torso and let the pleasure wash over you as you both reach your ecstasy.

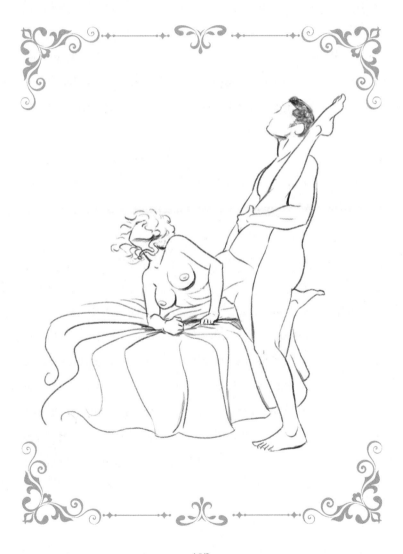

THE LOUNGER

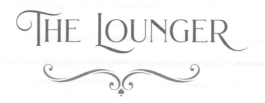

Cast your cares aside and cross your legs for a truly decadent tryst. Lie on your back on a soft surface—whether that is in the luxury of your sleeping quarters or on a picnic blanket—and raise your legs for his arrival. Keep them parallel as he moves into you, and then cross them at the ankles or at the knees for an even tighter clasp around his shaft. Caress yourself so he can watch as he plunges into you—running your fingertips over your nipples and clutching your breasts when his every thrust becomes more than you can bear. Move your pelvis in tandem with his while keeping your thighs taut, and reach for his thighs or backside to help keep the fluid motion.

As this rapturous affair leads you to breathlessness, tighten your muscles around his penis in rapid succession. He will feel you close around him for an astounding fit, and you will be sure to hear your name in moans. As you firm up your vagina around him, feel the intensity of your pleasure fully and keep it steadily in sync with his plunges toward oblivion. You will ensure his undoing and you will feel your brimming pleasure overflow in waves.

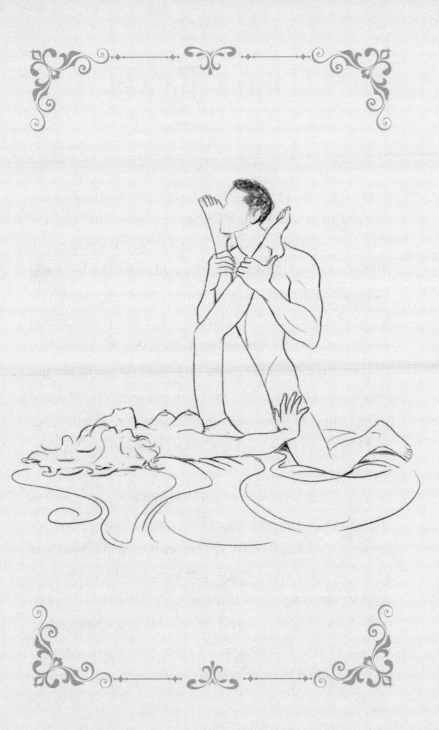

OPEN BOOK

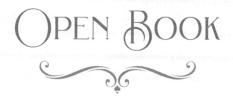

There is no end to the fantasies found upon opening a good work of literature, and here those fantasies come true. Let your pages flutter open for him as he uses his forefinger to scan what is inside. With your legs splayed wide, he should warm you up by encircling the inside of your vagina with his finger, changing direction every now and then but not letting up on pressure. Let him see the beauty that lies before him and caress your own curves for his benefit. When he can feel your wetness on his hands, have him rub your clitoris to send you spiraling. Look at him as he pleasures you, keeping your eyes locked so he can catch a glimpse of the sensuous universe he is about to enter.

When it all becomes too much, let him scoop up your legs and move into you with the ease he created from all that rich attention. As he holds your legs out wide, he will explore you profoundly. The angle of your hips will allow him to find the deepest parts of you, so be prepared to claw at the bed cushions with this feeling of powerful fullness. No doubt he shall lose himself in you, ramping up his speed with fierce abandon. Should you find yourself in need of extra attention to keep up with him, massage your clitoris in steady circles while he thrusts. The dual stimulation will build the way to your satisfaction and his.

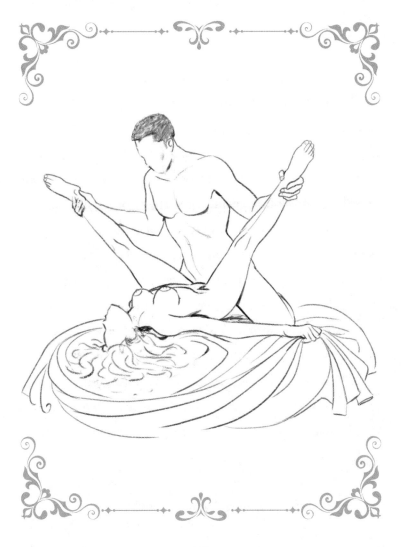

SWEEP ME OFF MY FEET

Lose yourself in love and lust with this sultry diversion. When coy flirtation, furtive glances, and stolen touches have you buzzing with excitement, you may just wish to forgo the tenderest of encounters in favor of something decidedly more salacious. Find yourself swept off your feet and onto your back, hugging your legs into your chest. Bring him to you, using your hand to guide him into your elegance. Place your feet on his chest and keep your knees closed to secure yourself around his shaft. Clench your muscles and watch his reaction as he feels your warmth surrounding him.

Hold on to one another's hips so you can keep the direction and intervals of his thrusts sure and true. Pull him toward you as he leans in and loosen as he recedes, keeping your legs against your chest all the while. When his speed overtakes you, lie back and let your arms fall where they may. Accept his love while keeping your hips engaged; if you can match his movement, propel your hips up to meet his thrusts. If you are dazed by the pleasure at hand, simply let it overcome you.

Call out to him—moan his name and let him know the whirlwind he has caused. Ask him how you feel to him and what he likes most. Encourage him with honeyed words or salty ones, and bring one another over the edge and into a most amorous oblivion.

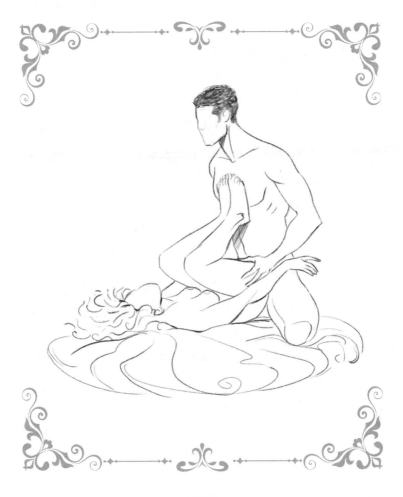

SWEET EMBRACE

Hold him closer in this most satisfying of encirclements. With your hips down and your legs aloft, you will pull him toward you and wish to never let him go. Place your feet on his shoulders, letting your toes rest delicately behind his ears. If your feet are sensitive, he can stroke your legs and softly kiss the inside of your ankles, running his tongue along your instep. As he brings his lips to these sensitive places, he should use his free hand to tease and tempt you even further. He can run his fingertips luxuriantly down the length of your thighs and press them into your vagina, rhythmically moving in and out to ensure you are more than just flushed at his touch.

When the time is right, pull him inside you and pull his body down close to you so your thighs are close against your chest. You should be able to feel him fall into you deeply. He may keep his pace slow and strong, taking agonizingly long strokes inside you to send your senses soaring, or he may pick up speed with force to leave you gasping for air. Should he perform the latter, you will feel his testicles rap against your underside in a way that accentuates your pleasure. Whatever your haste, be certain to gaze at one another as your bliss mounts. Connect in this moment of passion, and watch the lines of his face soften as your movements lead to his release.

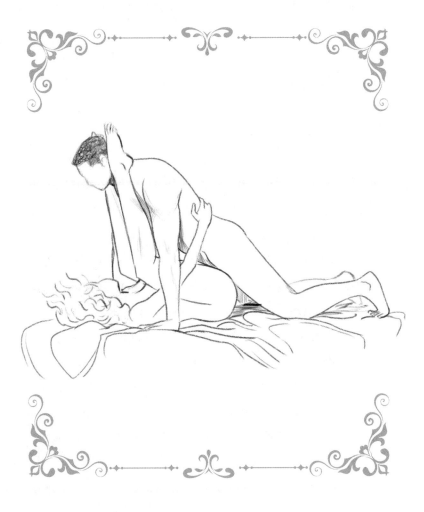

On Bended Knee

A gentleman's display of humble devotion may come in many forms, from a declaration to the queen attesting to the fortitude of your love to a desperate plea for forgiveness outside your front door. He might also get down on one knee. In this demonstration of love and generosity, he kneels on the bed and takes your legs in his arms, casting his gaze down to let his eyes wander across the landscape of your skin. To ensure that this is not just any ordinary bedroom romp, he should take care to tantalize you. Let him glide his penis along your vulva without inserting himself. As you become more wet from the thrill of feeling him close without fully having him, he will slide freely along you and feel your excitement against his shaft. Let him know how good this feels and engage in a playful game of temptation.

When the teasing has gone on long enough and he succumbs to your pleas for satisfaction, take him inside and squeeze your muscles tightly as he plunges into you. Now is the time for his alacrity—encourage a strong and swift pace so all the tension you have built up can be satiated thoroughly. Move your hips eagerly along with him, and as you both come closer to climax, wrap your legs around his waist and pull him down to you. Bring your arms around him so you are tightly wrapped—this will allow him to feel you more deeply and also press him against your clitoris. Brace closely as he shows you the love you deserve and you both achieve your bliss.

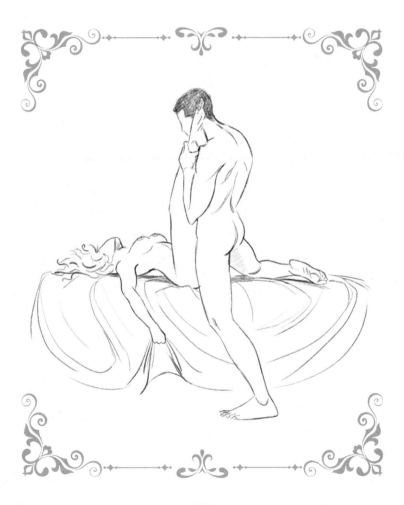

THE FOUNTAIN

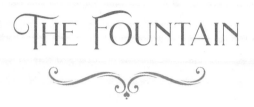

In expressions of love there is always beauty and in expressions of lust there is rapture, and this lovely encounter has both. Forgo the propriety of high society and find your satisfaction in decidedly impolite ways. In this steamy scene, you slink your way onto all fours and let him take in your magnificence from behind. As he strokes your skin and grabs your hips with sureness to bring you onto him, keep your arms steady and your body nimble. Extend a leg behind you to rest above his bended knee, and open your hips so he can drive farther into you. Engage your leg muscles to hold firm around him, locking your pelvis with his so you can move fluidly together. Keep your arms agile and your hips open as you let your love flow.

Should you begin to tire, keep your passions burning by bringing yourself upright so he can hold you close and you can continue to move along his shaft. Let him use his strength to move you up and down, cupping your breast as he goes. If you are looking for even deeper penetration and to tighten your grip around him, lower yourself onto your forearms instead so your pelvis is angled down and he can lean more profoundly into you. Pick up your speed and prepare for your hunger for one another to be generously sated. Invite your most libidinous desires into this scene and let your bodies move unrelentingly toward euphoria.

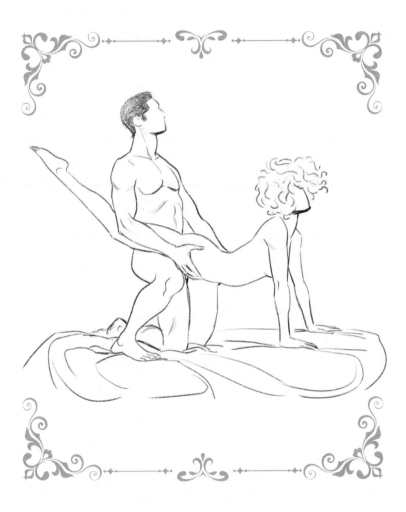

Entirely Devoted

Responsibility sometimes pulls a duke away from his duchess for fortnights at a time. When his coach pulls up and he returns to the warmth of your hearth, he may need to make up for lost rendezvous. In this luxuriant scenario, let him show you the devotion you had been missing after time away from one another. On a bed or a plush couch, lie back and stretch your arms so your back arches and your breasts perk up. Ensure that your back and neck are supported against a cushion or edge of the bed so you can bask in the pleasure you are about to receive. As he kneels on the bed and clutches your legs to spread them, hug your thighs against his hips to hold on to him.

Let him glide into you with the intensity of a man who knows just what you need to make you blossom. As he moves into you, have him rub your clitoris while you lengthen your body to intensify the sensations. When your passion powers up, he may move down on top of you or bring you up to him to carry you by the hips. Clutch around his neck to bring yourself closer, allowing your clitoris to rub against him and giving you more command over his pleasure. Keep up your breathless endeavors and use the closeness to kiss each other's necks or vocalize your desires. Ramp up your pleasure until you can no longer contain your composure.

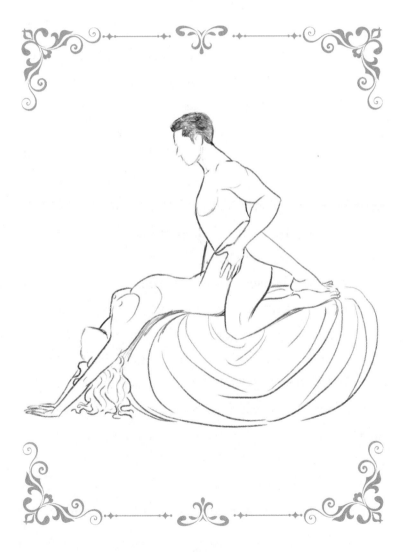

THE GARLAND

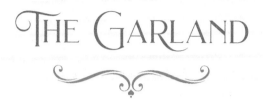

Love is in bloom in this sensational pose. Drape yourself across your partner's hips in a seated position, keeping your back straight and your legs in a squat. Lower yourself onto his shaft and prepare to flourish. Place your hands on his chest or biceps for leverage as you move atop him, quickening your pace for steady bursts of pleasure. With your hips open and your knees turned out, he will be able to discover the deepest part of you. As you move atop him, he will have perfect reach of your breasts. Let his clutch keep you excited and yearning to feel him more insistently.

You are in command of this encounter, but you can decide whether he gets to lie back and be astounded by your intensity, or if he should do his part to earn this amorous honor. This steamy stance requires both earnestness and endurance. If you begin to tire, have him hold your hands with a strong grip so you can press down on him for leverage, or have him sit up for a short period so you can cling breathlessly to one another and slow your haste. When you are ready for release, return to the original pose and let the passion overtake you. Keep your momentum quick and even until you reach your pinnacle.

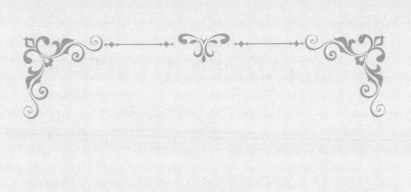

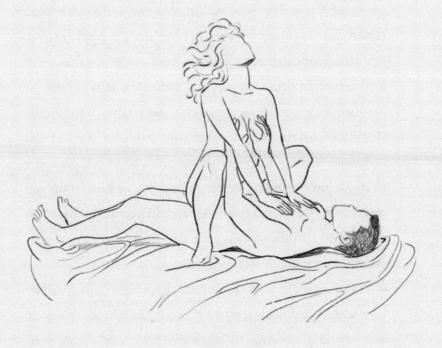

GARDEN GATE

An impressive flowering archway is an essential accent to any green of Grosvenor Square, but this one is found behind closed doors. Not for the faint of heart nor the rigid of spine, this scandalous dalliance presents itself at the confluence of lust and confidence unique to voracious new lovers. If backbends are not in your repertoire, this is best left to fantasy. Begin by readying one another with seductive caresses and passionate kissing. Let your desires run wild so you are eager to climb him. Standing before each other, let him scoop you up so that he remains standing tall and you wrap your legs around him. Slide down onto his shaft and begin your ravenous undoing of one another.

When you are ready to impress, have him unfold you by leaning forward while supporting your back. Arch your spine and extend your arms to reach the floor. Make sure your hands are planted evenly on the ground, and keep your legs around his waist for support. As he moves slowly in and out, feel the rush of intensity and let it send your body buzzing. When it becomes too much—and it surely will—bring yourself upright to cling to him as you climax, or lower yourselves gently to the floor so you can ravish one another with abandon.

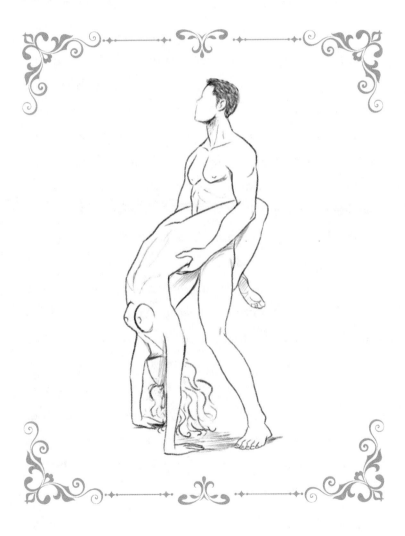

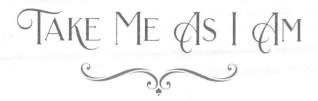

TAKE ME AS I AM

Let your naked desires reveal themselves in a position that demands intensity. Lie on a bed or cushioned surface, and let him come to you on his knees. You will want to be nimble and burning for this pose, so have him warm you up with the soft touch of his eager tongue. As he encircles your clitoris and whets your appetite, relax your limbs and feel the pleasure wash over you. Run your hands through his hair and whisper your longings as he sends thrills up your body. When you become desperate to feel him inside you, coo him closer and sit yourself up on the bed.

As he plunges into you, he should pick you up by the hips to carry your bottom and steady your body. With his knees spread apart for robust foundation, he can move into you with wildness. Keep your arms unlocked so you can move with him, and squeeze him tight with your muscles so his pleasure is multiplied. When you need to catch your breath, lower your arms and body to the bed so your hips remain aloft but your torso is supported. Play with your tempo at this time—slowing down to a tantalizing pace so he can take the time to rub your clitoris and tease you, or ramping up the speed so it is unrelenting and sure to end in gasps for air.

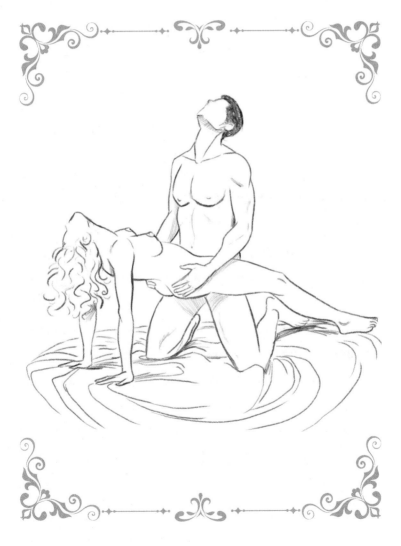

BURN FOR YOU

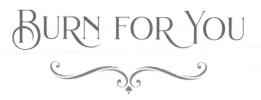

Some fires run hot, others smolder over time, and some are kept at bay until they burst into a wild conflagration. In this fiery tryst, you can finally yield to your yearnings like never before. Climb up your partner and have him carry you to a sturdy surface where he can rest one foot, like a step or a coffee table. Drape your arms around his shoulders and legs around his hips, using his raised leg for support. Look deeply into one another's eyes and feel the flames that brought you together.

Invite him inside you and tighten your legs to bring him as close as you can. He can use his raised leg to help lift and lower you onto his penis, or use his strength to lift you with his embrace. Kiss one another deeply, taking breaks to catch one another's gazes. Keep your back straight and your stomach close to him so you can enjoy the position longer. When the feeling of him moving in and out of you begins to overwhelm you, wrap your arms even more tightly around him and use the sweat of your bodies to continue your glide into euphoria. Tighten your muscles to empower your excitement, and show each other just how much your love burns.

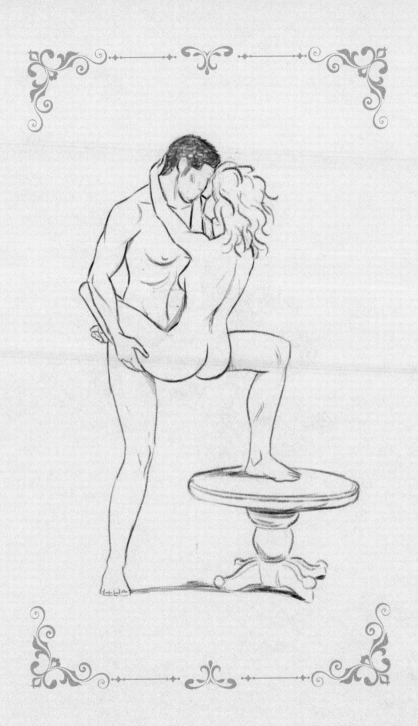

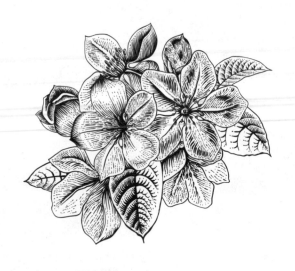

THE
INSPIRATION

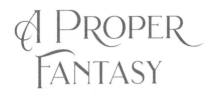

A Proper Fantasy

IS YOUR IMAGINATION POSITIVELY HUMMING with prurient possibilities, dear reader? Now that you have a most salacious education, you may allow thoughts of Grosvenor Square's most lascivious encounters to occupy your mind and stoke your flame. Taking one's sensual inspiration from *Bridgerton* is simple—there is so much to be admired, attempted, and enjoyed. But perhaps you wish to explore those most scandalous scenarios and delectable characters more *directly*.

The alluring content in this section attempts to help you not only fine-tune your favorite *Bridgerton* fantasies but also bring them to life in all their vibrant, candy-colored glory. For it is the erotic among the elegant, the lecherous among the chaste, that make these stories so scintillating. Whether you prefer to simply recreate some of the steamy scenes between beloved characters or to step into their exquisite slippers and stylish riding boots entirely, you will surely find innumerable ways to enhance your entanglements.

Don Daphne's innocence like a gracefully tailored dress

and bring propriety to bed with you. Assume the role of the rakish duke and have your way with your partner in a secluded garden. Get so carried away with your desire that you utilize the nearest desk, dressing room, or tree for your activities. It is time to put some of the tantalizing tips you have discovered among these pages into practice!

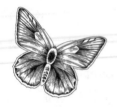

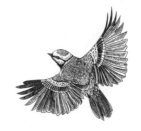

CHAPTER 8

Spontaneous Romps

DESPITE SIR HENRY GRANVILLE'S ASSERTION that delicious debauchery exists only on his side of town, sensual encounters seem to lurk around every corner in Mayfair. Entanglements are not just the mandatory purview of married couples—they are something to be reveled in as often as possible and whenever the mood should strike! Spontaneous romps may not always be practical amidst the bustling hum of our modern *ton*, but you may be able to find more opportunities for them than you imagine.

This chapter shall help you hone in on your *Bridgerton*-inspired desires and encourage you to take such opportunities where you may. Relish a free-spirited frolic in the garden or take a libidinous break from work. Keep your amorous efforts covert or scandalize passersby with your passionate moans. Whatever romantic path you choose to take in life, do be sure to embrace the unexpected and seize each sensual moment with your love. The prudish standards of high society need not dictate your private (or mostly private) encounters.

A PICNIC FEAST

Having one's own castle on an incredible expanse of manicured land would certainly prove useful in finding spots for spontaneous midday romps. Without a second thought, Simon and Daphne are able to push aside their beautifully

MAGNOLIA
Message: Love of Nature

There is nothing so striking as the graceful beauty of a magnolia blossom, except perhaps the sweet fragrance that lingers in the air about them. Magnolias were often gifted to women in appreciation of their gentleness, femininity, and beauty. Although that is a noble use of the magnificent magnolia, one could be a bit more intentional with its message. These beautiful blooms also symbolize a love of nature. Leave one for your lover to hint at outdoor encounters to come.

packed picnic lunch and feast on one another with only the wildlife (and perhaps a footman or two) to see. Would that we could all have that freedom—and that libido!

You may not have the privilege of doffing your clothing in the midst of a picnic lunch, but you can certainly turn the excursion into an appetizer for a more private affair. Pack a basket full of sensual foods—berries and cream, figs with honey, fresh oysters, and rich chocolate desserts would all do—and bring it to any patch of grass with an enchanting view. (Choosing a public park may, in fact, add to the intrigue.) Sit with your limbs entangled while you eat, using your fingers to feed one another. With the taste of something delicious still on your tongue, kiss your partner deeply. Then head home and see if you can make it out of your car before having your way with one another.

A MONUMENT TO YOU

Again, owning pastoral property in Regency-era England certainly had its perks when it came to adventurous entanglements. Dotting one's land with stone structures seems to be especially helpful for times when the skies open up unexpectedly. These monuments might serve as a stage for a gentleman to declare his love, or simply as a dry surface for newlyweds to use to quench their voracious thirst for one another.

In lieu of a concrete temple, you might use a secluded carport, porch, or even an open deck for your rendezvous. Whichever area you select, make sure you wait until darkness and sleep have settled over your area so as not to scandalize any wakeful neighbors. The sexy key to this type of entanglement is enjoying it quietly. Leave a trail of clothing behind you as you make your way to your chosen spot. (You may, however, wish to grab a blanket as you go.) Then—as near to silently as possible—devour each other with the night air touching your bare skin.

SERIOUS BUSINESS

Few things can unfurrow a brow as easily as a swiftly enacted seduction. Simon's mood certainly improves after forsaking his tenant worries for a few minutes between his bride's legs. It is not just the break from one's burdens that makes this sort of entanglement so appealing. It is also the immediacy of your lover's need for you. To allow your lust for your partner to push important things from your mind is quite the compliment to them.

When next you find your partner feeling anxious or concerned, set out to take their mind off their qualms. Like Daphne, place yourself between your partner and their work. Try to tempt them away from their work with your kiss. Should they be receptive, deepen your endeavors. Whether you use your desk or the kitchen counter, the sofa or the floor, allow yourselves to be overcome by your desire right there. No matter how hasty the break, it will surely aid in relieving any tension your partner may feel.

AN ELEMENT OF SURPRISE

We cannot control the weather. But in the case of a warm summer rain, that is certainly not a bad thing. The smell of it on freshly cut grass, the sounds of crickets and birds chirping away in the twilight, the feeling of the water as it hits your bare skin—these things can all add to a sensual experience should you have the privacy and presence of mind to enjoy them.

The next time you get caught in the rain, do not rush to get indoors. Take a moment to let the water fall over you and your partner. Feel it on your face as you kiss. Imagine it

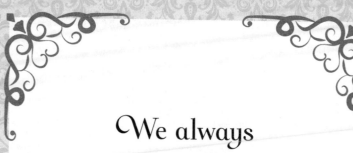

We always

long for the

FORBIDDEN

things, and

DESIRE

what is denied us.

—FRANCOIS RABELAIS

running down your bodies to all the places you wish to go. Let the water wash away your inhibitions and tell your partner how you feel about them. Only then may you make haste to get inside, carrying the sensuality of the water with you. (And if you should want the feeling of water on your skin *during* your activities, do not discount the luxurious sensation of embracing in a hot shower!)

ON THE STAIRS

Stairwells have an enchantment all their own on the residents of Grosvenor Square. From our own duke and duchess's lusty mid-conflict encounter to Benedict's first meeting of his own *amoreaux*, Madame Delacroix, at Sir Granville's bacchanalian soirée, they do seem to be the place for passionate embraces. Take a page from both stories and use the stairwell however it may suit your immediate needs, from fervent kiss to memorable encounter.

The stairs may not be the most comfortable of spots for a spontaneous rendezvous, so unless you are as hasty as our main characters, consider nabbing a pillow on your way up. But you need not stay in the stairwell for it to have its intended effect. As with Benedict and Genevieve, the stairs could simply be your initial stop. On your way up to the bedroom or down into the crowd, stay just long enough to transform your spark into a roaring flame. Then carry on with your evening, either dousing it presently or letting it burn until you can.

UNDER THE STAIRS

From meeting backstage with the dressing-room door open to reuniting under crowded bleachers at a public boxing event, Anthony and Siena's exploits do prove a bit riskier than is strictly prudent. That makes them hard to match, especially in today's privacy-starved society. Of course, should you want to be as adventurous as that passionate pair, you may still find ways to seek excitement without exposing yourselves to ridicule (or arrest).

The trick to courting scandal without being chained to it is to find a private venue in a public place—preferably one with a lock. An outlying study at a party swarming with guests would certainly do. Add an element of surprise by allowing your love to slip away first, then go in search of them. Should you feel guilty using your host's home in this way (after all, not all are as understanding as Sir Granville), there is no need to go too far. Simply sneaking away for a kiss may be all the thrill you need until you reach the comfortable privacy of your own bedroom.

RED GARDENIA

Message: Secret Love

Unlike so many red flowers, red gardenias represent a love relegated to secrecy. They also symbolize powerful attraction, making these seductive blooms an ideal gift for someone like Anthony to send to a certain opera singer on evenings when the call of high society kept them apart. Surprise your partner with red gardenias as a hint of passionate declarations to come, or as a nod to the initial spark of longtime lovers.

OFFENDING THE MAIDS

The mamas of the *ton* may disagree, but there is no shame in two consenting adults getting carried away with their passions … loudly. The maids of Clyvedon Castle certainly did not seem to mind their employers enjoying a lively honeymoon. In fact, noticing a couple appreciating each other's company could even be inspiring to some. So why not embrace your partner *emphatically*?

You may not have maids, but you surely have neighbors. Whether you share a wall with them or they are a mile away, try to forget they are there at all. Be as loud as you truly like, without reservation or concern that others may hear. Let your boisterous activities scandalize passersby. Most who do hear will either get a good chuckle from the sound or become motivated to make some noise of their own. And anyone who is so high in the instep that they find offense can have a seat with the likes of Cressida Cowper and let their envy consume them.

THE ROOSTER CROWS

Our lustful duke and duchess clearly feel they must seize every opportunity to enjoy each other's touch. We see them doing so practically morning, noon, and night and can imagine, with such a magnificent love match, that those habits extend well beyond the honeymoon. In fact, by keeping their flame high at all times, they ensure it continues to roar for years to come.

Stoking the embers of your love's interest in the mornings (and sometimes in the middle of the night) can certainly help you keep the flame alive. Can you think of a more alluring way to awaken than with your lover's kiss on your neck and their hand caressing you tenderly? When next you stir earlier than your partner, do exactly that. Keep your touch gentle and let your love's eyes flutter open before imparting your first kiss on their lips. When they begin to moan and move

Being deeply

LOVED

by someone gives

you strength,

while loving someone

DEEPLY

gives you courage.

—LAO TZU

their hands over your body as well, you can begin to seduce them in earnest. Together, you will set a happy tone for the day before you have even broken your fast.

ROUND TWO

Our duke and duchess clearly have a preference for fast and furious prizefights over the lengthy arias of opera. They tend toward the rhythm of a well-matched boxing event in the bedroom—several very sporting rounds leading, perhaps, to a final knockout punch. But even a knockout punch need not keep you down for long in this more enjoyable type of sparring, especially when you are as young and eager as these two.

Instead of seeing each sensual session as one and done, imagine they all belong to a longer encounter. This lets you pick up where you left off and opens you up to the possibility of enjoying each other more often, and in all sorts of circumstances. For example, when you have finished with your first round, you might retire to the shower (or a hot oil-scented bath). Once there, you run your soapy hands over your lover's body and they will not be able to resist returning the favor. Before you know it, a steamy round two has begun!

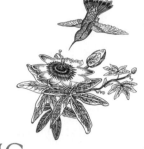

CHAPTER 9

AMOROUS INSPIRATION

AS LADY WHISTLEDOWN HERSELF would tell you, stepping into the slippers of another can be both exciting and liberating. How many of us have wished to be someone else, if only for a moment? Give yourself the freedom to act outside your own character—outside the bounds of propriety you have defined for yourself or have had defined for you—and you may reveal the possibility of even greater pleasure.

You are, of course, free to explore any story you may conceive of, but this chapter will give you a bit of sensual inspiration to start. Look to Benedict embracing his place as second son and allowing himself free rein to explore his creativity. Perhaps take the place of a favored couple and share in their fiery chemistry for a few moments. Whichever roles speak to you, step into them fully. You never know what you may uncover about yourself!

THE DUCHESS

Innocence can have its privileges. Allow yourself to be free from expectation, seeing your partner with only excitement and curiosity. Encourage them to take the lead and surprise you, but do not be passive. Instead, tease your partner throughout the encounter—perhaps even throughout the day. Be coy in your flirtation, bat your eyelashes (and perhaps a feathered fan, if you should have one), and allow yourself to be tempted ever so slowly. When you finally give in, do so completely, allowing passion to overtake you. And enjoy every kiss, caress, and thrust as if it is your first.

WHITE LILY
Message: My Love Is Pure

Symbolizing modesty, innocence, virtue, there could not be a more perfect flower than the white lily for our duchess. (Had her parents not resorted to banality in naming the children alphabetically, they might have considered Lily a much more suitable moniker for their first daughter.) Carry lilies as a reminder to meet every amorous encounter with the same astonished curiosity as our tale's heroine and you will be sure to enjoy them all.

THE OPERA SINGER

Acting as this sultry opera singer should be pure enjoyment! As Siena, you may use your wiles and lose your inhibitions. Dress in your most provocative ensemble and let your hair fall loosely around your face. Stare into your lover's eyes hungrily from across the room, then come together fiercely. Take control of your entanglement, kissing your partner passionately, using your body to move theirs, undressing them like you cannot wait a moment longer to have them. With Siena's wild and unrestrained energies, your activities may be quick, but they will certainly also be memorable.

THE GOSSIP

When you step into Lady Whistledown's very elegant shoes, do not think of her true identity's timidity. Think only of her commanding presence among the *ton*. You should wish to command control over your partner in the same tone—not in the eagerly passionate ways of Siena, but in the sense of someone who knows her own mind. Use your words (Lady Whistledown's mightiest weapon) to prompt your partner into scandalizing positions, perhaps even leaving them a lascivious note before your next liaison. But do keep your judgments to yourself—bruised egos do not belong in the bedroom.

Love and

Scandal

are the best

Sweeteners

of tea.

—*LOVE IN SEVERAL MASQUES*
BY HENRY FIELDING

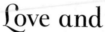

THE MODISTE

Like her salacious friend Siena, Genevieve Delacroix does not mince words when it comes to pleasure. She also offers you two equally delectable characters to choose from: the sophisticated French *modiste* who runs the most sought-after business in the *ton* or the open-minded reveler with the Cockney accent. Whether or not you test your French, you should don your best lingerie and your most seductive pout. Lead your love into temptation by the hand, the cravat, or whatever you happen to grab. Then demonstrate your adventurous approach by experimenting with a few of the positions in Part II.

THE COUNTESS

Lady Danbury hears all and is never wrong. This formidable woman is well led by her instincts, with impeccable timing and a sharp tongue that never fails to make her point. But hers is a quiet strength—she need not bark orders to be understood. Bring this spirit of knowing authority with you into the bedroom. Keep your head held high and be quite clear about your desires while you also tend to your partner's needs. This is not the same thing as taking control. It is simply *being* in control. And there may be nothing more alluring!

THE QUEEN

Queen Charlotte commands of her court not only respect but total submission. Of her husband, however, she desires only the warmth of his affection. You see how she softens in his presence. Which of these two sides you choose to portray is your prerogative as queen. Perhaps you start with an icy visage, letting your partner shower you into a more amenable state of mind with treats, compliments, and caresses. Once in the privacy of your bedroom, you may drop your defenses and treat your partner like your king. Either way, remember that *you* make the rules in this *ton*.

THE DUKE

The Duke of Hastings certainly gave us enough inspiration to work with. Rakishly insatiable but tender and adoring, Simon's is quite the gratifying role to step into. He feels the same hunger as the Viscount Bridgerton, but his is based in love and not temptation. Simon burns for his bride, always putting Daphne's pleasure first. To truly embody this incredible character, hold yourself nobly but give your partner that devastatingly sly, sensuous smile as you take them in your arms. And, of course, ensure you are creative in your endeavors, utilizing every staircase, desk, and stone temple in your possession for your spontaneous romps.

THE VISCOUNT

This Bridgerton brother balks hardest at tradition despite maintaining a fine and decent façade. For all his talk of being proper, he certainly seems to have a fixation on public displays of *affection*. But Anthony does not sneak—his entanglements are as wildly passionate as they are spontaneous. He attends to his hunger like a wolf stalking its prey. To personify the surly viscount, let your hunger overtake you wherever it may. Sweep your partner into your arms and consume them with a kiss. Let your need for them overtake you, and hopefully you will be met with equal fervor.

THE SECOND SON

The second Bridgerton brother clearly feels the pressure to conform, but his true nature is aching to break free from its constraints. Deep down, Benedict is an artist and an open-minded pleasure seeker. To embody his newly bold actions, you could host your own bacchanalia. You and your partner may wish to invite a third party into the bedroom, or you could enjoy each other among a home full of like-minded revelers. Should this be a bit much for your creative sensibilities, there is much sensuality to be found in simply sketching your lover's nude form before embracing it.

THE YOUNG TRAVELER

Like his sister, sweet Colin is pure of heart and looking for a true love match. He does not possess a drop of rakish blood. Instead, his doe-eyed nature, his innocent crush on Marina, and his ardent defense of his love to Anthony speak to him being a kind and affectionate partner. To embody the young Mr. Bridgerton, you must be tender and considerate toward your partner. See if you can elude their advances as well as he does Marina's. Then, when you finally give in, do so with the enthusiasm of youth!

THE ARTIST

Despite being perfectly respectable in the midst of high society, Sir Granville certainly enjoys coloring outside the lines in private. His encouragement of creativity, passion, and open-minded engagement is far ahead of its time but perfectly enticing in ours. Take from him the lesson of savoring the many pleasures of life. Go slowly and luxuriate in your

ENGLISH IVY

Message: Friendship, Fidelity, and Marriage

Ivy may not offer the silken petals or sweet scents of other flora, but it represents the very foundation of the successful love match. As a climbing vine, ivy must grip tightly the surfaces it clings to in order to grow. It is easily trained to move around obstacles, and its evergreen tendrils offer hope for the spring to come. With such admirable qualities, ivy is the most perfect plant to symbolize steadfast partnerships.

partner's touch, taste, and smell as you climb toward ecstasy together.

THE LOVE MATCH

To truly enjoy your entanglements as our favorite Mayfair residents, you must build a certain level of tension. Tempt your partner with suggestive actions, such as the licking of a spoon. Tease their skin with light touches throughout the day. And whatever you do, do not give in to your desires—not even a kiss. Allow the spark between you to grow slowly so when you do come together, you do so out of burning desire for one another.

THE SECRET LOVERS

The flame of some couples simply burns too brightly to last. That is the case of Anthony and Siena, whose ferocious passion for one another was more animalistic than amorous. That does not mean, however, that it cannot be enjoyable to embody every so often. When using these two as inspiration, conversation becomes unnecessary. Let high society fall by the wayside and tap into your inner animal. Kissing deeply, tearing off clothing, and vigorous activities are all encouraged.

THE TRUE PARTNERS

Will and Alice Mondrich surely offer a partnership worth emulation. Their interactions are loving and respectful, proving their relationship is one between equals. And with Will's profession, we can only imagine their entanglements are rather athletic and exciting. This is a pair that holds conversation in high regard, so do your best to communicate your desires to your partner. The gentleman may use feats of strength, such as carrying his sweetheart to the bedroom. But, true to Alice, she should be the one in charge!

Is one

expected to be a

GENTLEMAN

when one is stiff?

—MARQUIS DE SADE

On the Ladder

Never in your wildest dreams could a rendezvous on a ladder be so intoxicating. You may find yourselves perusing the bookshelves of your own magnificent library, or perhaps this affair occurs during renovations to your estate. When you have grabbed the book you were after, you can get down from that ladder—or your partner can just go down on you. Position yourself with your back to the rungs a step or two above the ground so you are above him. Lean back and let him do the work. Kiss each other passionately and let your hands roam free. As he moves down your body, kissing slowly until he reaches your softest parts, you can run your hands through his hair or brace his shoulders, or just hold on tight to those rungs behind you.

Keep your back aligned with the ladder, and if your knees start to get weak from his tongue rhythmically encircling your clitoris, move your feet to the floor for stability. As he builds your passion, he can move away from the clitoris and move his tongue in and out of your vagina, or he can use his hands to fill you while he tongues you down. As he brings your bliss to its brim, he can stand and enter you to feel your orgasm around his shaft. This could bring him over the edge as it might a certain duke, or it could lead to a standing romp so powerful that you are treated with a second peak.

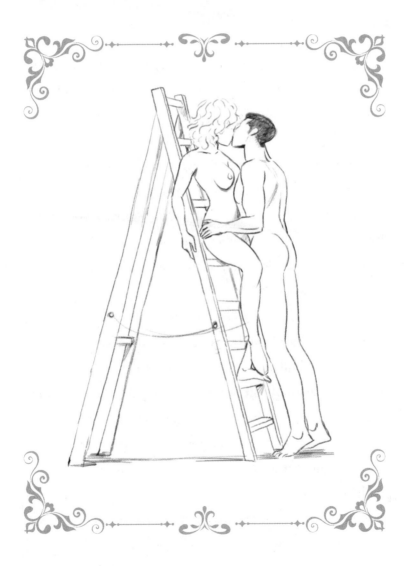

PERENNIAL LOVE

A walk amongst the trees can bring epiphanies for some and euphoria for others. When you find your natural proclivities taking over in a natural setting, give in to your desires and let the world melt away. For this standing position—which can also occur indoors—let passionate kissing become primal in the fiercest of ways. Grasp and clutch one another, as if this moment is stolen and someone could interrupt you at any interval. Undress each other with your hands and unravel each other with your mouths, moaning when it feels good and clawing when it feels better.

Lean against the surface behind you and raise a leg to wrap around his hip and welcome him inside you. To begin, use this leg to pull him against you over and over as he thrusts. When your gasps for air become more rapid and your pleasure more desperate, let him scoop you up so you are fully off the ground and both legs are wrapped around him. He should use his strength and his hunger to continue moving into you with unyielding haste, and you can use yours to meet his movements. Get lost in this most natural of moments, and discover the ecstasy that comes with wild abandon.

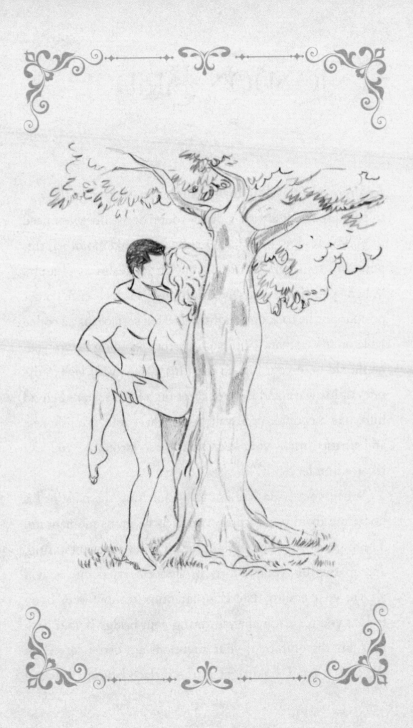

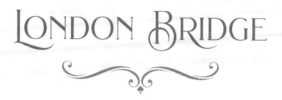

LONDON BRIDGE

As any world-traveling man of high society knows, the way to paradise is not always a direct route. Sometimes you need to build a bridge. In a steamy connection like no other, this pose will transport you to an uncharted realm of pleasure. When you find yourselves longing to feel each other profoundly, lie back on a slightly elevated surface, like a coffee table or an ottoman. With your partner standing before you, he should raise your hips to meet his. Drape your legs to the sides of his waist and rest your feet on a high surface behind him, like a counter or a wall. As he parts your exquisiteness and thrusts inside you, keep your torso strong so you can receive him fervently.

When your hands are not busy clutching the table or his body, use them to pleasure yourself as he gains momentum. The angle of your hips high in the air will have you buzzing, and massaging your clitoris in smooth, rapid circles will elevate your ecstasy. Pay close attention to how your body feels as you glide together, lowering your bridge if your back feels any discomfort. If your attentions are better served on the task at hand, hold tight to the surface beneath you and begin to tighten your muscles that surround him. The steady rhythm you create around his penis will be an indulgence for you, and a spur toward rapture for him. Feel the thrill of a new kind of liaison that will turn your world upside down.

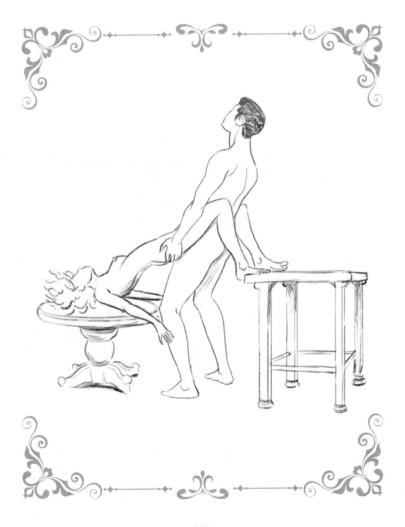

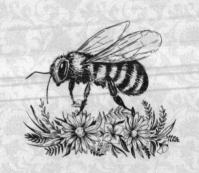